Bipolar Disorder
A Patient's Story

Bipolar Disorder
A Patient's Story

by

Charles Shelton

ISBN: 978-1-7336235-3-7

Dedication

I would like to dedicate this book to anyone who suffers from
bipolar disorder or any other form of mental illness.

CONTENTS

Acknowledgments

I would like to thank my family and my brothers and sisters for the encouragement and support that they have provided throughout my life in general.

And, most of all, thanks be to God for all the wonders of his creation, and the marvelous demonstrations of his enduring love.

Preface

The reason this book was written is to provide a personal, firsthand report, as well as a true narrative on what it is like to have and to live with bipolar disorder. And because it was written by a bipolar patient, you will be hearing and learning from someone who actually has the disorder, rather than getting secondhand information from someone who doesn't know what it's really like to have the illness.

What makes this written account so unique and wonderful is that because of the stigma that is associated with bipolar disorder, many who suffer from it are often too embarrassed and afraid of opening up or coming forward to talk about it. For them, it is just too taboo of a subject to openly admit that they have the illness, let alone talk about it, out of fear that they may be misunderstood, mislabeled, abandoned, or unfairly and adversely treated by others.

In addition to openly speaking about bipolar disorder, this book also offers real comfort, encouragement, and hope to other victims of the disorder, and to their families. It also serves to educate the public in regards to the real truth behind bipolar disorder. And helps to allay fears, and prejudices, as well as clear up certain misunderstandings, wrong teachings, and negative viewpoints about those who suffer from the often debilitating illness. The writer also shares some very encouraging, valuable, and useful things that have helped him to successfully cope and deal with major depression.[1]

Finally, this book goes beyond the surface, as it examines the root cause of bipolar disorder. And an intriguing theory is considered and proposed as to what may actually cause the illness.

Charles Shelton

4 July 2019

---

[1] This book is not a substitute for therapy.

Introduction

I was feeling all too strange, as I walked through the revolving glass doors at the hospital. I felt as though my mind was going to completely slip away from me! As I slowly moved through the doorway and into the lobby, suddenly, I felt like I just couldn't go any further, and that I needed to sit down. Luckily, there happened to be some chairs stationed there a short distance away from and directly facing the front door. So I immediately walked over and I took a seat.

Oddly and inexplicably, as I sat at the chair, I proceeded to glance back at the doorway. And when I did, I saw a most horrific sight! There were two women coming through the revolving door. The shocking thing is, the completion of their skin was chalky-white! the whitest white I have even seen! They looked like ghosts! And they had no eyes! but instead, in the socket areas where their eyes should be, there was large, round holes, that were pitch-black! Like charcoal. As the women passed by, they turned and they stared directly at me. What a frightening sight!

After the women left the area, I once again looked back at the front doorway. And when I did, I saw two paramedics wheeling a dead man on a gurney. They were entering the hospital through a standard doorway that is located right next to the revolving door. The weird thing is the dead man's body was lying uncovered and positioned in an upright sitting position of about a 45° angle on the stretcher.

As the paramedics wheeled the dead man pass me, I thought to myself: *"Wow... that sure is a strange sight! Why in the world are they bringing him through the front door and lobby of the hospital? This isn't the emergency room! But not only that, the guy is dead!"*

Suddenly, turning to my right, I looked and I saw a doctor walking and moving towards me in slow-motion. He was fully dressed in blue surgical scrubs, with a cap on his head. And he was wearing protective booties over his shoes. As he passed by, he slowly turned and he looked straight at me. And then he gave me a very weird and chilling, eerie smile! I thought to myself: *"Oh no! It finally happened! — I think I lost my mind!"* And then, immediately, I began to feel extremely suspicious. For some reason, I felt that everyone there, within the vicinity of the hospital, knew that I had gone crazy, and that they were just waiting for me to outwardly show it, so that they could grab me, and quickly whisk me away to a nuthouse or something.

Panicking, I immediately got up and left the area where I was sitting. And I entered a men's bathroom nearby, so that I could hide. Moving quickly, I entered the bathroom stall, and I sat down on the toilet, but with my pants still pulled up. I actually didn't have to use the bathroom. I was just there to hide. Because I didn't want to get caught by anyone that I felt might be looking to find and get me!

Initially, when I first entered the bathroom, there was no one in there except for me. But then, suddenly, two men came in, which only served to heighten my fear!

Although I couldn't see who the men were, I could hear them whispering something to one another. However, I couldn't make out what they were actually saying. The bizarre thing is; and I don't know how I knew this (because I couldn't see them from where I was hiding), but one of them was a white man, and the other one was black. Still feeling paranoid, and not knowing what to expect, I sat there motionless and in silence, and then they eventually left.

After the men were gone, I promptly got up and exited the bathroom. And then I walked over to and sat back down in the chair that I was initially sitting at when I first arrived at the hospital. I needed to sit down, because I was not feeling well.

As I sat there in the chair, a large and steady stream of people began to pass by. And then, suddenly, my wife appeared with our five year old granddaughter. But for some reason they didn't bother to stop or say anything to me. They just continued walking pass me.

The strange thing is, when my wife walked by, she turned and she looked at me, but then she quickly turned away. In response to her reaction, I thought to myself: *"Why is she ignoring me? Could it be that she realizes that I've gone crazy, and now she is afraid to be near me?"* Whatever the case, I felt that this was proof or confirmation that I did in fact, lose my mind.

I was both frightened and confused! I didn't know what to do! So I just continued to sit there in the chair for a moment. But then, afterwards, I quickly got up, and I followed after my wife and granddaughter, who were still walking and getting further away... Luckily, after having lost sight of them for a moment; looking up and into the distance, I was able to regain sight of them. They were entering an elevator. But by the time I got there, I missed it. So I waited for the next one to come.

As I waited at the elevator door, a small group of people who were traveling together approached and stood by me. And when I turned and looked at them, I was completely shocked and taken aback! The reason being is because all of their faces were freakishly distorted and scary! So I quickly moved away from them and left the area. But, as soon as I walked away, I immediately got caught up in the flow of a large group of people who were walking through the hospital. And because they were pushing and pressing against me, I just went along with them, moving with the flow of the crowd. What a rush! I felt like I was floating down a river... being helplessly swept away by a raging torrent!

As I sheepishly and subjectively moved with the flow of the crowd, I became increasingly nervous and frightened, thinking that I was going to end up being pushed along and into an area or place where I didn't want to go. But, most importantly, I was getting too far away from where I needed to be, which was upstairs on the second floor with my wife and granddaughter.

Suddenly, the moving crowd that I was in, happened to pass by an in-house café and coffee shop. So I quickly mustered up the courage and strength that I needed to push my way out of the flowing herd of people. And I jumped in the food service line of a long and growing line of customers who were waiting to be served at the restaurant.

As I stood there waiting in the long, food line, it gradually got smaller and smaller, until finally it was my turn to be served. Subsequently, the restaurant's service counter girl, a young lady, smiled and looked at me, and said: "What can I get for you, Sir?" In answer, I said: "A cup of coffee please." Afterwards, I paid her; took the coffee; and then I walked over to and sat down at one of the café tables nearby.

As I sat there at the table, I was becoming increasingly frightened, paranoid, and confused! I didn't know what to do! I sensed that I was in a lot of trouble! But I was just too afraid to show or give any type of hint or sign to anyone that I had gone crazy or mad. Because I was fearful that if someone was to find out, that they would come and take me away and lock me up in a madhouse.

Sitting there, I tried my best to look normal, so as to blend in with everyone else. I attempted to take a drink of my coffee, but my hand was shaking so uncontrollably, that the coffee started to spill out of the cup. So I placed it back down on the table.

Suddenly, my legs started to grow numb, cold, and weak. Initially, the numbness began in my feet only, but then, it slowly and gradually started working its way up my legs. I was not feeling well at all! The truth is I was in desperate need of help! But yet, I was too afraid to ask for it! What a dilemma!

As I sat there, people (other customers) began congregating all around me. Some were sitting at tables nearby, and others were coming and going. One person was a doctor, dressed partly in surgical scrubs and civilian clothes, who proceeded to walk over to and help himself to some condiments at the coffee shop condiment station nearby.

Because I was feeling both paranoid and afraid, I didn't know who to trust! Finally, after I remained sitting for a while, a middle-aged woman walked by me. And because I now realized that I could no longer put it off, and that I was in desperate and immediate need of help, I finally mustered up the courage to ask her for assistance. I simply had no other choice! Because I was feeling all too strange, and the numbness in my body was only growing and getting much worse!

Getting her attention, I said to the woman: "Excuse me, Ma'am. But, I'm not feeling well!"

"What's the matter? Do you have the flu?" the Lady asked.

In response, I didn't know what to say. And I surely didn't want to tell her the truth — that I had gone mad! So I said: "Yep."

"Do you need a wheelchair?" She asked.

"Yes," I replied. And then she quickly turned and left.

After the woman left, within a moment or so later, two men, who were hospital staff workers or volunteers or something, approach me with a wheelchair. In response, I said to them: "I don't feel well!" So they kindly assisted and helped me get into the wheelchair.

While I was being seated in the wheelchair, I could hear one of the female workers at the restaurant service counter say to her fellow coworker, concerning me: "Ooh, girl! I told you not to be giving coffee to just anybody!" Afterwards, I was quickly whisked away by the two men.

As I was being wheeled down a long hallway, I gave the two men my full name and address. I also told them the reason why I was at the hospital — that I was there with my wife and granddaughter. And that my wife is presently upstairs on the second floor, being given an iron infusion treatment, because her body is low of iron. The men didn't ask for or request this information from me. I just voluntary gave it to them. Because I wanted to project an image that my brain was still functioning properly, and that I was mentally sound, so as to try to convince or fool them into thinking that I didn't really lose my mind after all, when in fact I did. Afterwards, I was quickly taken to the emergency room.

No, as much as I would have liked it to have been, this was no mere dream. Nor was I having a nightmare. It was all so real! Later, I found out that I was experiencing a panic attack, along with a psychotic episode.[2] Also, I was told that I am bipolar, something that I was completely unaware of — that is, up until that very weird, strange, and unforgettable day. Little did I realize it at the time but my life was about to drastically change.

---

[2] Fortunately for me, after this one and only time, I haven't had anything like this happen since.

Chapter 1

BIPOLAR DISORDER

U nfortunately, in the year 2010-11, I was diagnosed with bipolar disorder. I was 54 years old at the time. What is bipolar disorder? Bipolar disorder, formerly known as "Manic Depression," is clinical depression, a mental illness. This type of depression is much different and more severe than the ordinary, common or garden variety depression, the regular, normal ups and downs of life.

One prominent characteristic or feature of bipolar disorder is that it involves two distinct and separate phases of mood swings, that alternate between prolonged episodes of an overwhelming sad state of depressive lows, to manic highs. In other words, a person with bipolar experiences severe mood swings that go from depressive lows, to euphoric highs.

As respects bipolar disorder, there are two main types. They are: "Bipolar I," and "Bipolar II." Both are mental illnesses. However, it is important to note, that although patients with

Bipolar I, and Bipolar II experience mood swings, there is somewhat of a slight difference between the two groups or categories, as noted below:

Bipolar I: The symptoms of Bipolar I, consists of a sequential cycling that alternates between two severe mood swings, both low and high. They are: (1) the "Depressive Episode," and (2) the "Mania Episode," with at least one episode of full-blown mania in a person's lifetime. Mania meaning: Euphoric or great excitement, marked by hyperactivity.

Bipolar II: This is similar to Bipolar I. And yet, it is somewhat different. Its symptoms include a vacillating or alternating between two separate and different mood swings, which are: (1) the "Depressive Phase," and (2) the "Hypomanic Phase," that never erupts into or reaches full-blown mania, which is more severe.

An interesting fact to note is that the mood swings associated with Bipolar I, and Bipolar II, are not like a light switch that quickly turns on, and then off again. These phases or episodes may last for up to weeks, or even months at a time.

Bipolar Depressive Phase

Speaking from experience, I can honestly say that bipolar disorder is one of the worst, if not the most difficult and painful thing to live with.

Often, in my case, the bipolar depressive phase is an extremely sad and hopeless feeling, type of state—a sort of deep and gnawing, emotionally painful sadness, that consumes, overwhelms, and eats at the soul. At times, it can be so extremely anguishing, distressing, miserable, and intense, that it makes you groan, and even weep and cry. During this time, you feel like your heart is shattered or broken, or like you're mourning the death of a loved one, but only ten times worse! And it can be so physically, mentally, and emotionally draining that you don't even have the energy, desire, or strength to go anywhere or to do anything. Often, all you want to do is sleep.

Along with producing agonizing and tormenting internal pain, bipolar disorder can also kill your emotions, and also your will or desire to do things, even things that you may have thoroughly enjoyed in the past. It can leave you feeling empty and lifeless inside, making your heart insensitive, unresponsive, or non-expressive to natural feelings such as love and joy that normal, healthy people regularly have and show. At times it can be so overwhelming that it's virtually impossible to even muster up a smile.

Due to the unrelenting sad and overwhelming degree of emotional pain that's often associated with bipolar depression, it can cause feelings of hopelessness, that perhaps your heart will never ever feel true joy and happiness again. You look for comfort and seek relief, but these things seem to have vanished from off the face of the earth. At times, things can get so bad, that you loathe your life, and you wish that you had never been born. You feel like the man of ancient times in the Bible, whose name was Job, who because of his unceasing misery, pain, and sufferings, cursed the day he was born. (Job 3:1)

Some well meaning people may tell the bipolar patient to just snap out of it. However, bipolar depression is not something that can just simply be willed away with a positive outlook. Like cancer, diabetes, or some other chronic disease, bipolar disorder is an illness. The dark moods of depression are beyond the sufferer's control. They cannot force themselves out of it. Unfortunately, for the most part, they are simply left with no other alternative, but to let it run its painfully disruptive course.[3]

Speaking from experience, at times it feels like the only way for the sufferer to gain possible relief from the misery and pain, would be to just lie down and die; which is something that I have often prayed and hoped for in the past. It's not that I would

---

[3] Although, the dark moods that are associated with bipolar disorder are beyond the sufferer's control, with the assistance of medications, and other forms of treatment, which I will discuss later, these can often help one to better cope with the often debilitating illness.

actually kill myself (although at times the thought did enter, and then quickly leave my mind); it's just that I didn't want to live like this anymore. Luckily, my will to live for both me, and my family, and also my love, hope, and faith in God is stronger than taking the so-called easy way out.

What about medications? Can they help? Yes, prescribed medications can be helpful in treating bipolar disorder. But the truth is, they cannot bring back the past, making you healthy and "normal" again. For the most part, they often mask the pain, leaving you feeling numb. However, this can be better than not receiving any help at all.

Because bipolar disorder can be so painful and difficult to personally cope and deal with, there are times when you need people to show you that they care—those who are willing to sympathize with you and comfort you during your time of need. But, sad to say, many times you don't get the understanding and support that you desire and need, but instead, people avoid you, or treat you unsympathetically. What's surprising, is that I can honestly say that I am not angry or upset with them for acting or behaving this way, because unless they themselves have experienced what it's like to be bipolar, how are they to really know and understand what you are actually going through. Also, due to bad publicity and the stigma that's often attached to bipolar disorder, many are simply misinformed. Thankfully, in my case, I have a very supportive and loving wife and family, which helps tremendously!

Bipolar Mania Phase

In addition to the bipolar *depressive* phase, there is also the *manic* phase, which is the flipside of things, at the opposite end of the bipolar spectrum. Although, with 'Bipolar II' the hypomanic stage never reaches full-blown mania; with 'Bipolar I' the manic phase can cause a euphoric, excited and energetic state that can foster excessive physical activity, and even make one feel superhuman.

During the manic phase, a person seldom needs rest and sleep, because their mind and energy level is on maximum overload, being pumped up and on the constant go! Often, when other "normal" people are sleeping, a person in manic phase might be up all night working on a project, or be on their hands and knees cleaning every inch of the house with a toothbrush so to speak. Interestingly, this euphoric phase can go on for days, and even weeks at a time.

One time, when I was undergoing a manic episode, I painted and redecorated — non-stop — the entire interior of our huge, three story, rental home, which at the time my wife and I were sharing with our daughter and her children. The house had six bedrooms, three full size bathrooms, a large kitchen with seating area, a formal dining room, a big family or entertainment room, and more.

As it turned out, in the end this gigantic painting project winded up costing me a pretty penny—a small fortune. Because, even though we didn't own the property, I decided to personally pay for all of the paint myself. The reason why, is because knowing the home owners or landlords thinking or mentality, I knew that if we were to request that the interior of the house be painted, that they would squawk in complaint, and refuse to pay for the paint and labor costs of having to contract a professional painter to do it. But even though this was the case, I still desired to have it done. Sure, the cost and work that I did was a lot; however, in the long run it paid off. For putting a nice, fresh coat of paint on the walls, along with adding a little colorful and decorative décor, enhanced our home's dull appearance, thereby providing a more uplifting environment for me and my family to live in. But, most importantly, it gave me something to burn all of my dynamic, manic energy on.

The thing that is most interestingly about this large painting and redecorating project, is that I worked hard at it for several days, nonstop, with very little to no rest at all, until it was completely finished. And then, after this, I went on to work on another big project.

When it comes to the *manic* and *depressive* stages of bipolar; the crazy thing is, if I could choose which one I would prefer, I would choose to be in the manic phase all of the time, rather than having to cope and deal with the painful depressive phase. However, as good as this might seem, in reality, this too is unnatural and abnormal behavior for a person.

Racing Thoughts

One notable symptom or feature that comes with manic depression is that one's mind often races out of control. While normal, healthy thinking usually consists of moderately paced, deliberate, and structured channeled thoughts that follow a certain or particular directed path. With bipolar patients it is often different. For example, in my case, I often find that my mind rapidly changes from one idea or thought to the next. This makes it very hard to focus and concentrate on things, and also to listen to other people when they are speaking, etc. And then, there are times when my mind is racing so not stop and fast that I can't shut it down, not even to get needed rest during bedtime. Luckily, if it wasn't for sleep inducing medications that are used to combat this, there are nights when I wouldn't get any sleep at all.

Hypersensitivity to Sound and Light

Another symptom of bipolar disorder is that one's ears can be overly sensitive to noise. Often, the tiniest, little sounds can be amplified many times over — some sounding like gunshot blasts! This can be pretty startling, especially if they occur randomly or are totally unexpected. Personally, when I'm at home, I often have to wear ear protection (the heavy duty kind of ear muffs that are normally used at a gun range) to muffle out harmful and annoying noises and sounds. Other times, when I happen to be out and about in public, and I am in need of relief, I prefer to wear ear plugs inserts, which are not as noticeable.

In addition to the ears being highly sensitive to noise, another annoying thing is that bipolar disorder patient's eyes can be extremely sensitive to lights.[4]

Having to deal with hypersensitive ears and eyes can make being in social gatherings and crowds very challenging. For the most part, I try to avoid them as much as possible, because it's so easy to become aggravated and annoyed. I don't know what causes the human body to react this way, but when you think about it, usually, when a person is sick or ill their senses often have a heightened sense of feelings and sensitivity—in that their vision, hearing, taste, smell, and touch become overly sensitive. Whatever the case may be, some of the symptoms that I mentioned above, which often and unavoidably come with bipolar disorder, seems to confirm that it is in fact an illness.

Bipolar Facts

How many people suffer from bipolar disorder? According to a National Institute of Mental Health (NIMH) report, "An estimated 2.8% of U.S. adults had bipolar disorder in the past year." That's roughly about 9.2 million people within the current United States population alone. Interestingly, in some people bipolar disorder has been diagnosed early, when they are in their teens.

Who are susceptible to getting bipolar disorder? As it is, bipolar disorder shows no distinction. It does not target any one type of person or group in particular. Both males and females are equally affected, no matter what age, race, ethnic group, or social class they may belong to.

What causes bipolar disorder? Although, there are some thoughts as to what might cause it, as it currently stands, it is

---

[4] Although there are additional things, the things listed above are just some of the symptoms of my mental illness. Also, as respects other bipolar patients, they may experience similar symptoms, or they may have some symptoms that are different than mine. The same is true respecting the degrees of intensity. Some patient's symptoms may be more or less intense than others.

unknown.

Is bipolar disorder a genetic disease? Even though some indicators seem to suggest genetics may be involved, it still remains uncertain if this is an actual cause.

Do emotional traumas, or environmental conditions cause bipolar disorder? In some cases, emotional traumas have been known to trigger bipolar disorder. And as far as environmental factor or influence is concerned, it is uncertain as to whether this causes it. However, for some people, I personally believe that environment can and does play a significantly large role in one's developing bipolar disorder, which is a theory I will attempt to prove later in my discussion. But, of course, I will leave it up to you the reader to decide, once you have considered all of the presented evidence and facts.

Is bipolar disorder curable? Unfortunately, the answer is no. It is a chronic disease. But the good news is it is treatable. Some of the things that are often used to treat bipolar disorder are: Medications, Psychotherapy, and Electroconvulsive Therapy (ECT), things which I will now briefly discuss.

Prescribed Medications

There are a variety of medicines that have been developed over time to help treat bipolar disorder. There are mood stabilizers, antidepressants, and anti-anxiety medications.

As it stands, bipolar medications like any other healthcare medications are prescribed by a doctor. In this case, it is a mental health professional or clinical physiatrist who prescribes them—based upon the patients needs and the effectiveness of the drug. It is his or her duty to properly evaluate their patient's medical condition and prescribe medications or treatments based upon individual need, medication effectiveness and success rate, and so forth—things that are not always easy to quickly diagnose and determine. The reason being is because it takes time to analyze and properly evaluate a person's symptoms and arrive at proper conclusions, which involves closely monitoring and evaluating their moods, behavior, etc., over an extended period of time. Also, what works for one patient, may not necessarily work for another.

Some of the medications that are used to treat bipolar disorder are: Prozac, Lithium, Seroquel, Zyprexa, Risperdal, and the list goes on.

Are there medication side effects for these drugs? Unfortunately, the answer is yes. What are they? Well, although side effects may vary per medication and individual, some common side effects of these medicines include: nausea, headaches, tiredness, dizziness, drowsiness, and weight gain.

One medication that I was initially given during the early stage of my bipolar illness, made me feel like a zombie. After a couple of weeks I had to stop taking it, and I asked my doctor to prescribe me something different, which he did.

Another medication, named Ambien, which I was taking for sleep, actually caused some very strange effects. Interestingly, this I would not have known if it weren't for my son Joseph,[5] and other telltale, visible signs.

My strange experience with Ambien was this: Late one night, about 2:00 am or so, Joseph (who was in his twenties at the time), and I was up watching TV together. Also, in addition to this, I was cooking some food on the stove. Okay, so what's so strange about these things, you might ask? Well, the strange this was, during the entire time, I was sleep walking!

The scary thing is, initially, at the time, both Joseph and I didn't know that I was actually sleepwalking. But, as time elapsed he began to notice that something just didn't seem right with me. So he awoke and alerted his mother (who had gone to bed earlier that night), about the strange situation. He said: "Mom, I think that

---

[5] The name has been changed.

Dad is sleepwalking!" In the meantime, I had gone back to bed, but in our guess bedroom.

The next day, when I woke up in the morning; to my surprise, I was quickly informed about what had happened to me the night before. However, not before I had discovered something else first. And that was, when I had awakened that morning, I was surrounded in bed by fudgsicles and ice-cream sandwich rappers. One ice-cream sandwich that apparently I was holding onto for quite some time, was even melted in my hand, which made a gooey and sticky mess.

The curious thing is, I don't know how many nights prior to this that I might have sleepwalked. All I know is that I had been taking Ambien for some time, and because I had recently and unexplainably been putting on a lot of weight, the evidence seemed to suggest that I was possibly sleepwalking and eating at night on a regular basis, for a considerable time period!

Later, I informed both my physiatrist and mental health therapist about my bizarre, sleepwalking episode, and they told me to cease taking Ambien immediately, which was a good decision, seeing that I could have hurt myself or others, or possibly, might have even burned down the house!

Help for Anxiety

Along with clinical depression, often comes the feeling of anxiousness. But there are also medications that can help with this too.

Some of the medications that are used to treat and reduce symptoms of anxiety associated with depression are: Ativan, Lexapro, Zoloft, Celexa, KlonoPIN, etc. Interestingly, new medications are becoming available all of the time. By the time this book is published and released to the public there will probably be others on the market.

Are there any medication side effects for the drugs listed above that are used to treat anxiety? Unfortunately, the answer is yes. Although, side effects may vary per medication and individual, some common side effects of these medicines include: insomnia, drowsiness, dizziness, and upset stomach.

Concerning prescribed medications associated with bipolar disorder, sometimes you feel a little bit like a Ginny pig or lab rat that is being experimented on, because doctors often have to change your medication or try several different kinds. Nevertheless, this is something that may be required at times, in order for them to be able to find the right medication that is best for you, because not all medication works the same for everyone. What works for one person may not work for another. Also, sometimes the medications that you may have been taking for quite some time, might eventually lose their effectiveness. And so you may be prescribed or given something else to take its place.

As with many things in life, with prescription drugs there are usually certain known side effects. And these may not always be the best or greatest to have to cope with or endure. But often, the positive benefits that the medications offer can far outweigh the negative experiences. The important thing for bipolar disorder patents is that once you begin taking your medications, it is important to stay consistent with them, for if you stop taking them, you can suffer a mental relapse.

Chemical Imbalance

It is a commonly held belief that people who suffer from clinical depression have a chemical imbalance in the brain. Interestingly, back in the year 1984, there was thought to be about thirty different types of known chemicals in the human brain. However, today, with more knowledge and research, it's been discovered that there are many more! And like many things in life, often, it is important to have a perfect balance in order to function properly or to be healthy.

Of the many chemicals in the human brain, one that seems to be notably off balance or low in volume in those who suffer from bipolar disorder is serotonin. Serotonin functions as a neurotransmitter, which helps to relay messages from one area of the brain to another. Subsequently, to help boost low serotonin levels in mental health patients, they are often prescribed antidepressant medications. An interesting thing is that, theoretically speaking, there is no way of truly knowing for sure what the proper, correct, exact, or normal levels of serotonin are or what they are supposed to be in the human body and brain—there is no way for scientists and those in the medical field to be certain. The reason being is that the human body and brain is just too complex! It is only by means of trials and experimentation that they have noted that by boosting or increasing the levels of serotonin in bipolar patients, that it seems to somewhat help in treating their depression.

Psychotherapy

Psychotherapy, is another alternative treatment that can be used to treat bipolar patients. Psychotherapy is talk therapy, which usually takes place between the bipolar disorder patient, and a mental health therapist. However, this is often offered in both individual and group settings, depending on what method is preferred by the patient.

The goal of the mental health therapist is to listen patiently to the patient's, allowing them to express their true feelings and concerns, and then to offer any suggestions that might aid in helping them to cope with their disorder. Also, the patient's are taught how to recognize when a mood shift is about to occur, so that they can be better equipped to handle it when it does arise. In addition, patients are also taught effective stress reducing methods and techniques.

Both individual and group settings for psychotherapy can be helpful. However, usually, when it comes down to it, it all depends on what a person's preference is. Personally, I've had both.

Interestingly, as far as group sessions are concerned, while personally attending them, I found other bipolar patients to be very encouraging and supportive, both to me and to one another. Also, it was very comforting to learn that some of them were actually going though some of the same problems or things that I was experiencing.

Electroconvulsive Therapy

Electroconvulsive Therapy (ECT) or "shock treatment" as it is sometimes referred to, is another form of treatment that can be used to treat bipolar patients.

ECT is a procedure that is administered under general anesthesia, which involves intentionally feeding small currents of electricity into the brain, for the purpose of inducing a brief seizure. Although, it is not fully understood how it works, it has been known to offer relief to some bipolar patients who suffer from debilitating depression.

"Electroshock therapy," as ECT was formally called in the past, was given a lot of bad news or publicly in 1975, with the highly popular and acclaimed theatrical blockbuster movie entitled "One Flew Over the Cuckoo's Nest," starring in the main character roles, actor, Jack Nicolson, as the mischievous and rebellious patient, Randle Patrick McMurphy, and actress, Louise Fletcher, as the mean and ironfisted nurse named, Ratched. However, ECT can be an effective form of therapy that can be helpful in administering needed relief to mental health patients suffering from debilitating depression.

Interesting to note, is that ECT therapy is a sort of last resort type of therapy that is usually warranted and recommended only when nothing else, such as medication, psychotherapy, and other things… don't seem to be working. Nevertheless, it is totally a personal decision to pursue.

At one time in the past, ECT treatment was actually recommended and prescribed for me personally, which I was even hospitalized to have done. However, later, during the preparation process, and with further consideration (based upon receiving more information about the procedure, and its possible side effects), my family and I, for personal reasons, decided that it was best for me to forgo the treatment at that time. Nevertheless, there are many people yearly that have ECT therapy treatments administered, and it has worked well for them.

Bipolar Myths

The following bulleted items below are some incorrect myths about bipolar disorder. They are:

- *People with bipolar disorder have mood swings that shift back and forth quickly, like the flip of a light switch.* (False) The depressive phase, as well as the mania (or hypomania) phase, can last for weeks or even months at a time.

- *Bipolar disorder people are insane or crazy.* (False) Interestingly, in talking with and listening to many people, I've noticed that the word *bipolar* is often synonymously used with the word *crazy,* when people are discussing, evaluating, or explaining a bipolar person's mental state; as if these two things are both alike in significance and meaning. However, linking these two things together, as though they mean the same thing, is totally incorrect. Because the actual medical definition of bipolar disorder does not mean that a person with this condition is crazy. It simply means that they suffer from manic depression. So to suggest or say that bipolar people in general are crazy is completely wrong. Bipolar people in general are not nuts or mentally deranged, but rather, they simply suffer from cycles of depression, and mania (or hypomania).

- *Bipolar disorder patients are violent people.* (False) Although, some people by nature may be overly aggressive or physical, this does not mean that all bipolar people are violent. In general, they are not monsters, or ticking time bombs lying dormant, just waiting to explode. Take for example United States of America President, Abraham Lincoln, who was bipolar. He was known to be a pretty mellow individual by nature. I couldn't even imagine him going ballistic on someone. He didn't even attempt to fight back when his half crazed wife, Mary Ann Todd Lincoln, frequently would punch, hit, and beat on him.

- *Bipolar disorder people are non-spiritual people that do not have God's spirit, approval, blessing, and support.* (False) One's spiritually and relationship with God has nothing to do with bipolar disorder. It is not a spiritual illness, but rather, it is a medical illness or disease.

If you happen to be a bipolar patient, or if you know someone who is, it is nothing to be ashamed of. For many people bipolar is a way of life, something that they learn to live with. As a matter of fact some of the most gifted, talented, creative, inspiring, intelligent, highly successful, influential, and productive people in the world, both past and present were/are bipolar, as the list below shows.

Famous Bipolar People:

Below is a list of famous bipolar people, both past and present:

- Vincent van Gogh – artist and painter.
- Edgar Allan Poe – poet and writer.
- Ernest Hemingway – writer and journalist.
- Charles Dickens – writer.
- Abraham Lincoln – American president.
- Florence Nightingale – founder of modern nursing.
- Mark Twain – writer and humorist.
- Vivien Leigh – actress.
- Kim Novak – actress.
- Marilyn Monroe – actress.
- Jimmy Piersall – Boston red sox hall of famer.
- Delonte West – professional basketball player.
- Mel Gibson – actor and director.

- Richard Dreyfuss – actor.
- Robert Downy Jr. – actor, and film producer.
- Judy Garland – actress, and singer.
- Patty Duke – actress.
- Rosemary Clooney – singer, actress.
- Rene Russo – actress, and model.
- Jim Carrey – actor and comedian.
- Maria Bamford – comedian.
- Linda Hamilton – actress.
- Carrie Fisher – actress, writer, comedian, activist.
- Catherine Zeta-Jones – actress.
- Jean-Claude Van Damme – martial artist and actor.
- Connie Francis – singer.
- Nina Simone – singer, songwriter, pianist, and journalist.
- Dusty Springfield – singer.
- Frank Sinatra – singer and actor.
- Charlie Sheen – actor.
- Jimi Hendrix – guitarist, singer and songwriter.
- Jaco Pastorius – musician, composer, and producer.
- Charley Pride – country singer, and musician.
- Kurt Cobain – singer, songwriter, and musician.
- Britney Spears – singer, dancer, and actress.
- Selena Gomez – singer, actress, songwriter, and producer.
- Sinéad O'Connor – singer, songwriter, and musician.
- Chris Brown – singer, dancer, and actor.
- Demi Lovato – singer, songwriter, actress, and model.
- Mariah Carey – Singer, songwriter, record producer, actress.
- Dick Cavett – television personality and former talk show host.
- Jane Pauley – television anchor and journalist.
- Ted Turner – Entrepreneur, television producer, media proprietor, and philanthropist.
- Jesse Jackson, Jr. – American civil rights activist and politician.
- Jonathan Winters – actor, comedian.
- Ben Stiller – actor, comedian, and filmmaker.
- Burgess Meredith – actor, producer, director, and writer.

- Francis Ford Coppola – film director, producer, and screenwriter.
- Winston Churchill – prime minister, and journalist.
- Theodore Roosevelt – American president.
- Ludwig van Beethoven – composer and pianist.
- Wolfgang Amadeus Mozart – composer and pianist.
- Virginia Woolf – Novelist.
- Rembrandt Van Rijn – painter and printmaker.
- Pablo Picasso – painter, sculptor, printmaker, poet, and playwright.
- Sir Isaac Newton – physicist and mathematician.

*Sources[6]

---

[6] For sources, see *"Sources,"* on pp. 248-254.

Chapter 2

THE ROOT CAUSE

OF MENTAL ILLNESS

Sometimes, it's not an easy thing to look back at and recount one's past, especially if there happened to be negative things or experiences in it that hurt us, caused us bad feelings, or brought us emotional pain, etc. However, sometimes facing one's demons so to speak is what is needed in order to release pent-up or suppressed anger or pain, which can be of great aide in helping one to get onto the roadway of healing and recovery. Also, there are times when we have to look back at the past in order to understand or make sense of the present, because what happened or took place in the past often lays the foundation for the future, or influences or creates what takes place today.

In this regards, I feel that doing a personal search for and finding the root cause of one's mental illness can also be tremendously beneficial. This is something that I did. It wasn't that someone suggested or told me to do this. It is just something that I personally thought about and chose to do on my own. True, it's not that finding out will necessary remove or take away one's illness, but at least it can help one to get to know their self better, and it can also help them to better cope with their disorder. But not only this, it is also important because it can help one to find and establish inner peace and contentment within themselves—things that are highly beneficial to one's overall health and wellbeing.

Interestingly, after finding what I believe to be the root cause of my mental illness, what I now have to say and reveal might seem a bit controversial to some, and it might ruffle their feathers somewhat (which is neither my wish nor intention. But, unfortunately, that's the way it is in life. Because some people will take offense at just about anything and everything you say or do), nevertheless, the truth of the matter is, it must be said or told. The fact is, a vital part of the natural healing process is not to hide or cover over things, but instead, to be able to openly and freely talk about and discuss the issue or problem with others.

I would like to clearly point out that I am no longer disappointed, angry, or anything about what has taken place in my life, or in the distant past, or what is occurring in the present. For I have comes to terms with it all. My main goal in reflecting on and delving into the past was to try to figure out and understand the reason for my condition or illness, so that I could possibly find a workable solution that would help me to make any necessary personal changes or improvements in my life so that I can better understand and cope with my bipolar disorder. This way I can perhaps get a hold on it so that it is not as debilitating and crippling, so that I can possibly go on to lead a much better and more productive life. Interestingly, one additional good thing that comes out all of this, is that with the valuable insight and knowledge that I've gained; perhaps this information can be of use to help others too who are undergoing similar problems or issues.

In retrospect, looking back at my past, if I had known back then, what I know today, I could have spared myself a whole lot of grief, heartache, and pain. But, as it is in life, that's not necessary how things work. In reality life is our tutor or teacher. And we must learn valuable lessons and experience many things along the way, both good and bad. There's no getting around this inevitable and truthful fact. However, on the flipside of things, along with the negative or bad experiences, life has also taught me many good and valuable things too, which are not only beneficial to me, but also are things that can be used to aid others — informative information that can be utilized to help them to understand certain things or to get through difficult or tuff times.

Before I begin explaining what I believe to be the root cause of my illness, might I caution, that if you also happen to be one who suffers from bipolar disorder, and you too decide to conduct a personal search to find the source of your illness, and you eventually discover what it is (which will most likely be different from mine, as well as others, for each of us are separate and distinct individuals), then the next step is to quickly come to terms with it, and then release it and let it go. The reason being is because you wouldn't want your findings to cause or stir up in you any possible feelings of resentment or hate towards others. This would only make matters worse. Your personal and private investigation should primarily be for the purpose of helping you to better understand yourself, and also to help you to better cope with your illness. Well, with this having been said, the following is what I found in my personal search.

Source of My Mental Illness

I am a person of mixed-race. I was born in the year 1956, in the city of St. Paul, Minnesota — the child of an interracial marriage, during the time of deep seated racial prejudices, dissention, and segregation in the United States of America, when the African-American Civil Rights Movement (1954-1968) was in full swing.

My father, Charles Shelton Sr., whom I was proudly named after, was both of African American and Native American decent. And my mother Kathryn was French and Irish (or Caucasian). Interestingly, as a result, from society's standpoint, I was considered "Black" from the moment of birth, although I was mixed or multi-raced, and also fair skinned in complexion.

Now that we have gotten this preliminary information out of the way, I will now go on to disclose or explain what I believe to be the root cause or main source of my clinical depression. The following is what I discovered.[7]

In searching for the root cause of my illness, I had to travel back in time, to a time long before I was even born, to the time period of institutional black slavery in North America, and to something in particular that happened back then that drastically altered or changed the character or image of the black race in general.

You may wonder or ask: What does slavery and what happened back then have to do with you being bipolar? Well, as it turns out, a whole lot. Let me explain.

Slavery in America

Black slavery in North America began in the year 1619, after groups of white men voyaged or traveled from America by large ships to the continent of Africa, where they then hunted, captured, and kidnapped native people of the land, and then brought them to America to sell them in the infamous slave trade.

Over the succeeding years and throughout many decades to follow, after many conscientious, deliberate, long, and arduous journeys — sailing over the vast and perilous Atlantic Ocean, thousands of miles round trip to Africa and back — millions of slaves (men, women, and children) were captured, transferred to America, and then sold into slavery.

What an utterly sad, shocking, and devastating, life altering experience this must have been for people of the African race to

---

[7] Although this information was initially intended to be for me alone, I later decided to make it available for the general public as well, in hopes that it might be of use to help others too.

have lost everything in a matter of an instant of time! Their poor lives were completely uprooted and shattered! And they would never be the same—no, never again! Many of them were not only cruelly torn away from their homes and families, but they also would never see or be reunited with their dear loved ones again!

Given a New Identity

Shorty after arriving in North America, the African people were given new names—each of which corresponded to their individual slave owner's name that had purchased them. But, before this they were also given something else, something that never in their wildest thoughts or dreams would they have ever imagined; something that would undeniably haunt and torment, not only them, but also their offspring and future descendants for untold centuries to come. What were they given?

Consequently, as it turned out, the African race (who was now on American soil) were given a completely *new identity* or *image* by their captors. You might ask: What image was it that they were given, and why?

Well, from the very moment the people of the African race stepped foot in America, and from that time forward, they were no longer looked upon as being intelligent human beings; as one of God's unique, beautiful, and wonderful earthly creations—his crowning achievement that was part of the human race, which as a whole is comprised of a large, multinational, multilingual, multiracial, worldwide human family.[8] No, but instead, they were severely downgraded in character value. Why? The reason why is because their captors, the perpetrators of slavery, knew that their true identity or image had to be drastically altered or changed in order for them to be accepted in their new role as slaves. For if they were introduced into the "New World" as normal human beings, as being equal in stature to whites (which they were), their

---

[8] The Bible explains that all humans were created in God's image. (Genesis 1:26-28) This means that all humans have or were given the divine attributes or qualities of love, wisdom, justice, and power.

plan to enslave and work them like lowly beasts would never have gotten off the ground.

In addition to the above information, because the white populous in general were undoubtedly unfamiliar with the African race prior to their arrival into the New World, the perpetrators of slavery also knew that they had to give the Africans an identity or image that was so hideous, grotesque, and brutish that it would serve to desensitize the hearts and feelings of America's white citizens, in regards to the slave's miserable plight, pain, and sufferings. This way they would be unlikely to show them any pity, sympathy, understanding, compassion, or mercy, in regards to using them as slaves, and in treating them unjustly and inhumane.

So, what image were the people of the African race given, and how was this accomplished?

As it turned out, the perpetrators of slavery used *slander*, or as I call it "character assassination," to destroy the people of the African race's true character or identity.[9] They did this by falsely and intentionally portraying and introducing them into the "New World" as being an ignorant, dumb, and brutish type of creature; one that was highly inferior to the white race in intelligence, which of course was a blatant lie.[10] Yes, the African race was deliberately vilified, horribly disgraced, and grossly disfigured by their captor's, although in actually there was nothing wrong with their

---

[9] Slander means: To smear, tarnish, defame, or vilify. Slander or "defamation of character," as it is often referred to in a legal sense, is a very serious offense. It has been compared or liked to actual murder. Because it can completely kill or destroy one's good name, reputation, and character. An example of this is what happened to people of the African race during the time of slavery. Interestingly, although it played a substantial role, it wasn't so much the slave's skin color that caused them to be mistreated, hated, and abused. But instead, the main reason why is because of the "false image" that they were given. And until the false image is completely gone or removed, the black race, who have inherited the image from their ancestors, and who today is often discriminated against, will continue to struggle for justice and equality.

[10] For proof that blacks are not inferior to whites, see the information "The Farce Openly Exposed," in Appendix A, on pages 238-240.

character or physical appearance. What a gross misrepresentation! Even a lowly dog was viewed and treated more humane! Unfortunately, this demoralizing *"False Image,"* as I have coined or call it, which was given to the black race, would go on to torment them, their offspring, and future descendants for untold centuries to come.

Far Reaching Effects of the "False Image"

What effect would their new identity, the "false image" have on the African people? Well, the fact is, the "false image" would not only serve to enslave them, but it would also cause them and their children an enormous amount of suffering and pain—emotionally, mentally, and physically. But, not to them only, for it had far-reaching effects.

Unfortunately, because the "false image" has been promoted and kept alive throughout American history by means of discriminatory practices aimed at blacks, and also wrong and misleading teachings about them as a people in general, it has gone on to haunt and torment the slave's future descendants for many generations to come, right down to the present day. For they (the people of the black race) have not been able to shake off or rise above the maligned character and distorted image that originally destroyed the true identity or character of their African ancestors long ago, a "false image," which they themselves have unjustly inherited. And that has greatly contributed to their being victims of modern day era's of oppression, racial injustices, segregation, and inequalities. As a matter of fact, it is the continued, unrelenting strong influence of the "false image" of the 'Negro' that fosters racism and discrimination against people of the black race today, and the very thing that keeps them from obtaining total equality. (For a concise list of the effects of the false image, see "Far-reaching Effects of the False Image," in Appendix A, on page 229)

You might say, okay, but what does all of this have to do with you being bipolar? Well, as it so happens, a great deal. Because this sad situation that transpired or happened in the past, is what laid the very foundation for the future environment that I would eventually be born and raised within, along with the thinking and mindset of the people in general—an environment and mindset that glorifies the "false image," and that often fosters discrimination and injustices against blacks.

Sad to say, it is this repulsive, negative, and destructive "false image" that I too have inherited from my ancestors—an image that both initiated and has continued to contribute much to my sufferings, emotional pain, and depression, as I will explain later in further detail.[11]

Why did the perpetrators of slavery and others commit this immoral and unjust crime against the black race? Apparently, it was all done for greedy financial gain (a plan that worked out perfectly and favorably for them, their offspring, and future descendants, as well as a large portion of the white race in general down to this very day). The fact is plantations were very lucrative and profitable industries that produced cotton, sugar, tobacco, coffee, and rice crops, etc. Crops that were all planted and harvested by *free manual labor,* which was a laborious and backbreaking type of work that was physically forced upon the enslaved African people.

So, in a nutshell so to speak, this is how slavery came to be in North America, and what it did to the image and lives of the people of the black race, both past and present.

The fact is slavery in America created an entirely different type of world for Africans, from the life that they were used to living back in their ancestral homeland of Africa. Undoubtedly, to them,

---

[11] It is important for me to note at this time that I am not bringing this matter or subject up in order to play the race card or to just harp on the injustices experienced by blacks. Neither is this information in any way meant to disrespect anyone or anything, especially the beautiful country of the United States in with I live. But rather, my soul purpose in this regards is to understand and explain the reason or root cause that initiated and contributed to my illness—Bipolar Disorder.

America was a cold and unnatural, strange world, that was dark and bleak—a place that was completely devoid of light, hope, and most notably love.[12] A world that was non-accepting of blacks, other than for the purpose of cruel slave labor. An inhumane world; an ungodly environment, where they were denied the right to live peaceful, joyful, productive, and healthy lives. It was a place that was filled with shattered dreams, broken hearts, and mournful souls—a life that crushed and destroyed all potentials for true happiness, peace, and prosperity, both individually and as families. It was an environment that bred and fed depression. (To note the effects of slavery on a person's spirit, see the box below.)

Effects of Slavery on the Spirit

What did slavery do to the individual slave?

- No doubt, it completely crushed his or her spirit.

How does one react, behave, and feel when they are mentally and emotionally crushed?

- They feel unjustly treated.
- They feel victimized, vulnerable, and powerless.
- Their feelings and emotions are deeply and negatively affected.
- They become sad and depressed.
- They feel self pity.
- They feel resentment and anger towards the people who treat or treated them wrongly.
- Their spirit becomes low.
- Their motivation is weakened.
- They feel like giving up.

Interestingly, if this mental and emotional crushing continues to systematically occur, the person is likely to eventually give up all hope.

---

[12] To see the effect that being loved (or not) can have on a person, see the information "Importance of Love," in Appendix A, on page 241)

The Struggle Continues

Although many centuries have passed since the initial days of black slavery, the menacing, erroneous "False Image" of the 'Negro' continues to wreak havoc. For this demoralizing and damaging image has gone on to negatively affect and detrimentally cost the black race in general all the way down to this very day.

Will the "false image," which has fostered racism and inequality towards black people ever be removed by man? Unfortunately, the answer is, it is highly unlikely. Why is that, might you ask? Well, for one, I have to agree with Albert Einstein who said: "No problem can be solved from the same level of consciousness that created it." But also, it is because the distorted "false image" of the black race, which was initially created through slander during the time of slavery, is too deeply imbedded in people's minds. And deep seated or sown images and prejudices are just too hard to overturn and erase. But also, it is because black slavery lies at the very heart or foundation of American society. The fact is, from the initial onset of slavery's establishment, which as an institution lasted for about 246 years in North America, it has become an integral part of the internal makeup or fabric of society. In other words, it is part of the inescapable daily social environment in which we currently live and breathe. (For further information on this, see "The Foundation of America," in Appendix A, on pages 218-222)

What makes matters even more challenging and difficult for the black race, is that a particular environment or system was intentionally created and established before and after slavery's abolishment in 1865, that was designed for the purpose of keeping the black race in a subservient and inferior position, as respects the white populous in general. It was a system that intentionally discriminated against people of the black race; one that made it extremely difficult for them to rise above and out of the pit of oppression, inequality, destitute, and despair. (For more information on this, see "The Black Codes, and Jim Crow Laws," in Appendix A, on pages 223-228)

Advancements Towards Racial Equality

Some may say: "But hasn't the black race in general made significant advancements in recent years towards achieving racial and social equality?" True, the black race in their fight for social justice and racial equality has gained a certain measure of progress in some areas. For example, in time, certain laws have been implemented for relief against discrimination in public accommodations, voting rights, equal employment opportunity, and so forth, such as "The Civil Rights Act of 1964," which outlawed discrimination based on race, color, religion, sex, and national origin. Also, "The Civil Rights Act of 1968" that proposed equal housing opportunities, etc... regardless of race, creed, or national origin. Nevertheless, as good as these and other laws may have intended to be, many people have seen and learned through experience that the application or enforcement of them is not necessarily automatic. For they often have to put up a hard fight to have them enforced. Also, these laws have not brought about total equality for the people of the black race in general, nor have they ended racism.

Some may point to the fact that the U.S. had its first black president, and suggest that this indicates substantial progress for black people in the matters of racial and social equality. But, in reality, does this alone prove that the black race in general has finally achieved it, and that disparaging discriminatory practices and racism towards them as a people are now things of the past? What do the facts show?

Well, although I'm sure that he meant to do good, the fact of the matter is, having a black President (2008-16) has in itself done little to nothing to stem the tide of racism in America; nor has it done anything substantial to equal or level out the playing field for them in the matter of achieving total racial and social equality, thereby effectively improving the lot and life of the black race in general. In other words, having a black president in the history books looks good, but in real life it didn't work as well as perhaps intended.

Some say that he was too busy sweeping things, like obvious racial disparities and prejudices under the rug. One way in particular, was by unwisely talking and acting as though racism is a thing of the past and that it no longer exists. Others argue that it was a matter of him putting other priorities ahead of more important things. Whatever the case, little to nothing was accomplished to substantially help the black race to achieve equality during his eight years in office.

But, to be realistic, honest, and fair to him or to anyone else for that matter, the truth is, you really can't point your finger at or put the blame solely on one person, for although he had many supporters that helped him get elected to office, on the other hand, he also had many, even his own political constituents, who during his somewhat brief, and yet, significant tenure in office, had shown that they were not ready to rally behind and support some of the decisions and undertakings of a black president. So, in this regards, it could be argued that his hands were somewhat tied as to some of the positive endeavors that he may have wished to accomplish. But, whatever the case, this clearly substantiates the truth of the matter, that he, like any other imperfect human being, even though they may be a good or great person (one that's passionate, genuine, and sincere, with wonderful goals and ambitions); that due to the sheer magnitude of the insuperable issues they face, they often lack the true power and ability that is required to solve some of mankind's big problems, both past and present.

Interestingly, for some non-minorities, having a black president gave them the excuse to sweep racism under the rug, and falsely proclaim that they are not prejudice, when in fact they are. Neither are they for real change.

Others might argue and confidently conclude within themselves, that the black race is making progress, but that it has been progressively in small increments, over an extended period of time or years. Sure, it may be true that the black race has made gradual advancements towards equality over the years. But, the question is, why so little movement, over such a long of a period of time? What is it that is impeding substantial growth and real progress? Again, the answer is, it is the direct result of the damaging effects of the "false image," that initially destroyed the people of the black race's true character and identity long ago; an untruthful image, which has been bred, fed, and kept alive over eons of time, by means of discriminatory practices aimed at blacks, and also wrong and misleading teachings about of them as a people. But, are these the only things that have promoted the "false image"? What about our modern day?

Modern Day Teachings and Beliefs

According to the history of the modern day era of the 20th century, and on into this early 21st century, two additional things that have promoted the concept of the "false image," are the teachings that blacks are *genetically* inferior to whites, as far as intelligence is concerned, and also generalized, negative, racial stereotyping of them as a group of people. However, these things are really nothing new. They are just the reiteration of old tactics of the past being presented in a slightly different way.

Are Whites More Intelligent than Blacks? Yes, many say. The white race have inherited more intelligence than blacks.

William Bradford Shockley Jr., a winner of the Nobel Prize in physics in 1956, strongly asserted this to be true. He said: "My research leads me inescapably to the opinion that the major cause of American Negroes' intellectual and social deficits is hereditary and racially genetic in origin." In other words, he asserted that blacks are inherently born intellectually inferior to whites—that it is in their genes.

Another person, former professor of psychology, Arthur Robert Jensen (also now deceased) of the University of California in Berkeley, who was a leading exponent of the view that whites are biologically superior to blacks in intelligence, declared: "The number of intelligence genes seems to be lower, overall, in the black population than in the white."

As shown in the above quotes, these two highly educated and prominent men both strongly asserted that the black race is genetically inferior to the white race. However, this teaching couldn't be farther from the truth! For neither has it, nor can it be proven.

As a result of the storm of controversy over the alleged lower inherent intelligence of blacks, the National Academy of Sciences declared: "There is no scientific basis for a statement that there are or that there are not substantial hereditary differences in intelligence between Negro and white populations. In the absence of some now-unforeseen way of equalizing all aspects of the environment, answers to this question can hardly be more than reasonable guesses. Such guesses can easily be biased, consciously or unconsciously, by political and social views."

Racial Stereotyping. Another thing that has promoted the teaching of the "false image," in our modern day world, is damaging racial stereotyping.

"Stereotyping" is when people have a preconceived or fixed belief about a particular group of people. Unfortunately, when it involves one's ethnicity or race it is usually negative.

Speaking from personal experience, as a minority, when it comes to negative racial stereotyping, I have to say that it is highly frustrating and upsetting when people don't recognize or appreciate you for what or who you truly are, but instead, they view and treat you as someone or something completely different. For example, because a person is black or a minority, some whites automatically assume that they are uneducated, and so they treat them and speak to them in a belittling, condescending way, like they are illiterate or stupid. There is a term for this today; it is called "Racial Profiling." Sadly, this and other forms of racial stereotyping are often a daily experience that many people of the black race have to deal with. But what is even more disturbing, is when they completely deflate or diminish your character value, and treat you as a worthless, good-for-nothing soul.

Unfortunately, the "false image" of the black race is so strong that nothing seems to be able to release its victims from its tenacious, vice-grip hold. It doesn't matter how well a black person may conduct or deport themselves in society, or how well educated they are or become, or even how much money or expensive material possessions they may possess. In the end, they are often viewed only one way, which is unequal and inferior to the white race in some fashion or form.

The crazy thing is that some white people who are prejudice don't even recognize within themselves that they have a problem with racism—that they are racist. Instead, they attribute the problem solely to the black race. Some say: "'They' (people of the black race) are just being too overly sensitive!" And "'They,' have a knack or fault of attributing every negative thing that happens to racism, when in fact it has nothing to do with racism at all!"

True, every negative thing that occurs doesn't have to do with race. However, what about attitudes, viewpoints, and actions that truly are racist, but that are often downplayed and ignored because people happen to be blind to themselves and their ways, or they are just too stubborn to recognize or admit it.

One thing that makes racism difficult to recognize in ourselves is that it is an insidious disease—something that gradually develops and becomes well established before it becomes apparent. And then, once it becomes deep-seated, it becomes harder to remove. The truth is we can only change the person that we see in the mirror. And, if the image that we see reflected is an inaccurate or distorted picture of ourselves, then how can we make the needed changes for improvement?

Interestingly, when it comes to prejudice, some people claim that they don't see color. In other words, they are trying to convince others that they are not prejudice. Personally, I think that this is one of the most absurd and stupidest statements that I have ever heard. For who, in their right mind (except for those who are born legally blind) doesn't see color? Personally, I know that I both see and appreciate colors. For example, isn't a flower vase or floral arrangement that contains a well arranged assortment of different types and colors of flowers a beautiful sight? Interestingly, if the flower vase or floral arrangement had only one type or color of flower, this could in itself be a very pretty and attractive thing. However, when you add a mixture or variety of different kinds and colors of flowers, it adds so much more depth and beauty to the arrangement.

So when it comes to reflecting on and speaking about races or the color of a person's skin, I believe that the best thinking and attitude is not to say, "I don't see color," but instead, to love and appreciate people and things for their unique differences and beauty. For this wonderful gift or feature called *"variety,"* is God's generous and loving arrangement for adding a plethora of diversity and joy to our lives![13] (Acts 17:26)

Interestingly, many white people don't mean to be racist. As a matter of fact, the poor mislead ones may not even realize that they are thinking and behaving this way. The reason being is because they have become accustomed to seeing it, and they unconsciously have been systematically programmed to think and act this way from a very early age. On the other hand, there are those who do realize that they have a problem with racism, but they are too stubborn to admit it, or they just don't care enough to make needed changes. For these, there's nothing that we can do, but to hope that someday they will wake up and come to their senses.

When it comes to all of the various or different races of humankind, the truth of the matter is, no one race is better or superior to another. For all people are equal in God's eyes, no matter what their race, ethnicity, or nationality happens to be. In the Bible it says: "He [God] *made* out of one man *every nation* of men to dwell on the entire surface of the earth." (Acts 17:26) It also states at Acts 10:34, 35 that "God *is not partial*... but in every nation, he who fears him and practices righteousness is acceptable

---

[13] God is not partial or prejudice. In the Bible at Acts 17:26 it says: "He [God] made out of one man [Adam] every nation of men." In other words, all nations and races of people have descended from the first man Adam.

to him." For more information on the equality of races, see the information "The Farce Openly Exposed," located in Appendix A, on pages 238-240.

Self Inflicted Woes

In addition to erroneous teachings and stereotyping of the people of the black race, there are other things that have added to the problem and intensified the negative effects of the "false image." What are they, you might ask? Well, for one, many blacks within today's generation refuse to educate themselves, and then they turn around and ridicule and persecute those who try.

Another thing is that some blacks have unwittingly made bad choices as to how they project themselves in society. Instead of conducting and deporting themselves with dignity and respect, they choose to add further insult and injury to the "false image" of the black race by means of unsightly dress and grooming, and careless, ill-advised, brazen actions, and damaging speech, such as by affectionately calling one another the derogatory "N" word; wearing sloppy, sagging pants that often extend below the buttocks; and also by portraying themselves and fellow blacks as being ignorant, disrespectful, and violent in hardcore, gangster rap music videos and songs, and so forth. But, little do they realize, that these bad and negative things only help to further promote ignorance and division, as well as to glorify and enhance the hideous "false image" that was given their ancestors who were slaves, for the purpose of making them seem less than human— like uncivilized animals—an image that blacks today, as their descendants have also unjustly inherited.[14]

Sad to say, in the case of many of the African slaves descendants today, slavery has never really ended, because by personal choice, they prefer to still enslave themselves and others of their own race to the destructive "false image," by adding

---

[14] Might I point out that it is not just young people who might exhibit or set a bad example. Because there are also many adults that do the same.

further pain and damage to it. What a disgrace![15]

However, fair to say, concerning some misguided or wayward black youths; you can't necessary, completely fault them, for in some cases it has to do with a term that I have coined or invented, called FOPP (Fulfilling Other Peoples Prophecy).

FOPP is when an individual intentionally fulfills another person or group's advanced prediction or prophecy concerning them, as to how their situation, life, or future will turn out — whether good or bad.

With FOPP there is only one of two possible fulfillments or scenarios, and they are:

Scenario 1:

This is when a person overly desires and wants to please another person or group (such as a parent, etc.), in order to make them feel happy or proud of them. And so they reach out to become the person or thing that these ones are hoping for (even if the chosen profession, or life, etc... is not of their own, individual, and preferred preference). For example, one may say: "When I grow up, I'm going to be a fire fighter, because that's what my father is, and what his father was before him. And that's want my father wants me to be." And so they become that person in order to please their father — accommodating his wish or wishes, in regards to his son's choice of profession or career; even if this doesn't personally bring the son any true joy or satisfaction.

Scenario 2:

This is when a person knowingly or unknowingly fulfills another person or group's negative or bad prediction/prophecy concerning

---

[15] It's important for me to point out that just like any other race of people, even through some blacks are bad examples, not all are this way. The truth is most African Americans are good and productive citizens, as wells as positive role models for their children and others. But unfortunately, the few that are bad make it harder for those who are trying and want to do what is good and right.

them, as to how their situation or life will eventually turn out. But only, they (the person that is being unfavorably judged) do this out of anger and spite, just to hurt and annoy the negative fault finders. For example, Johnny (the person being unfairly judged) may say concerning his fault finders: "If they (the judges or predictors of his eventual outcome) mistakenly and unjustly view and treat me as being a bad person, or something horrible, which I am not — such as being a lazy good for nothing, or a criminal or thug, etc. Then I'm going to give them exactly what they want! I will become that person, just out of spite, so that I can irritate and hurt them even more!" And so Johnny deliberately squanders any potential good, talents or gifts that he may innately possess, and ends up throwing away his life, thereby becoming a victim of FOPP.[16]

Sad to say, for many people of the black race, especially young ones; due to society's negative viewpoint, unjust judgment and treatment, and bad prediction or prophecy concerning them and their future success, it has become the second scenario listed above.

Unfortunately, in the past, I have actually known some young black people, whose outlook and future outcomes were unduly and negatively influenced for the worse by others, such as teachers, neighbors, parents, peers, and even complete strangers who had an overly negative and critical opinion of them.

In order for a person to totally give up, stop trying, or self destruct, they would have to feel complete hopelessness. The problem is, due to the influence of the "false image," many in today's American society have placed an extremely low character value upon the people of the black race in general. They are often labeled a failure from the very start. They are not expected to succeed in life. Unfortunately, after awhile, this overly critical and negative viewpoint of blacks, along with the discriminatory environment, becomes so discouraging and frustrating to many that

---

[16] The name Johnny is used only as an example. It does not refer to anyone in particular.

they eventually surrender to self-doubt, and give up hope. The truth is, a person can only be emotionally beat-up and demoralized so much, before it eventually takes away their desire and will to fight.

The fact of the matter is, racism is an ugly thing. Not only is it highly contagious, it is also very destructive. It creates division and fuels hatred. It frustrates and impedes potential progress and growth. It causes low self esteem. It breaks hearts and crushes souls. It can even cause one to completely give up, surrendering to skepticism and doubt. It weakens families and communities. And it destroys love and hope.

Racism Begets Racism

When it comes to being a victim of racism, there is a need for one to exercise extreme caution and restraint. The reason being is that it can be so easy for one to allow the sufferings, mistreatment, and injustices that they experience to cause them to become bitter and prejudice towards the very ones who treat them unjustly — in effect, fighting racism with racism. This not only makes matters worse, but, in the end, stored up resentment and hatred can completely destroy ones potential, development, and life — thereby robbing themselves and even their families of peace, joy, and happiness.

Unfortunately, as a result of experiencing racism, there are many blacks that have become racist themselves, showing themselves to be no better than those who hate or discriminate against them.

Racism — Who's to Blame?

As respects human nature, there is an inherited imperfection and sinfulness in humankind. But there is also a quality for good. And although there are times when there is a real struggle to do what is right, for the most part mankind in general strives for improvements in life, both economically and socially. With this in mind, then why is there such an ongoing problem with racism? What or who started racism, and also what keeps it going?

When it comes to the matter of determining or establishing racism origin, some people may have the tendency to point solely to one particular race of people and accuse them of creating or starting it. However, I personally don't believe that racism can be solely attributed to one race of people alone, because all races, no matter what ethnicity or nationally, are guilty of it to a certain degree or in some fashion or form. Also, neither do I believe that it is a manmade invention. The reason being is that if something is manmade, it could be easily overturned and conquered, like so many other manmade things have in the past. However, when it comes to the problem of racism, it's just seems to be too solidly fixed, and almost virtually impossible to remove. Why is this the case, you might ask? Well, one reason is because of human imperfection and the struggle to do what is right. Another reason is that there is a powerful, invisible force that is stronger than puny man, one that is driving a huge wedge between people, and pushing them to war and fight against themselves. It is a bad spirit that takes advantage of human imperfections; one that operates and feeds on things such as: differences of race, ethnic and national pride, selfishness, greed, arrogance, and other human weaknesses — anything and practically everything necessary, so as to separate, divide, and conquer people.

Unfortunately, this never ending battle of fighting against the dividing forces and influences of racism that we as humans are up against, is a fight that we must never surrender to or give up on, for the moment that we individually or collectively as a group let down our guard and give up, is when we collapse and suffer a disastrous and ignominious defeat.

Elements Needed to Destroy the False Image

Is there anything that can destroy the "false image," and end racism? The answer is yes. But it would take divine intervention, and a lot of hard work and united efforts to accomplish it. But not only this, it would have to be initiated or come from the top down.

The first, vitally important step leading to correcting this major issue is that first and foremost, society has to fully acknowledge the issue of racism—that there is a serious problem that exist. And then, next, the second step is that they must be willing to openly discuss and talk about it. Not in a debate or argumentative type of spirit or way, but rather, in a calm, rational, and peaceful manner, with the goal or objective of the two sides (both the white and black race) collectively and unitedly working together towards a common solution that will help correct the issue, rather than sweeping it under the rug as society has done in the past, and continues to do.

Unfortunately, because racism is such a touchy and sensitive subject to many, those with authority who are in a position to do something about it, for the most part seem to be content with just turning a blind eye and deaf ear to it.

Why is it that society is unwilling to open up and consider this serious problem that is primarily affecting the black race? Perhaps, it is because they feel that its black citizens don't have a real or legitimate complaint or problem that needs to be addressed and dealt with? Or perhaps, it's because they don't deem its black citizens as being valuable or important enough to listen to and consider? Or maybe, it's because they have been hearing complaints from blacks about this same issue for so long a period of time, that they have grown tired, and so now they just tune them out, hoping that it will just fade or go away? Or perhaps, it's because they simply just don't care? Interestingly, when it comes to different issues (even controversial ones) that are happening to other people in society, they are readily willing to discuss and deal with these things. But for some reason, when it comes to racism and problems affecting the black race, they are often intolerant, and unwilling to listen to and discuss these matters. However, until society or those in authority are willing to open up and consider these important issues, nothing will be done to change or correct these ever pervasive and ongoing problems.

The fact is, in order to completely eradicate or remove the "false image" (that has fostered today's racism and inequality towards black people), the structure of society as a whole would have to be completely uprooted, torn down, and replaced. Just a few changes, alterations, or a little patchwork here and there on the stained and torn fabric of society is not going to be enough to work. The *entire* fabric or structure of things must be uprooted and discarded. And then, afterwards, an entirely new and completely different arrangement or system of things needs to be designed, built, and put into place — one that will be just, equal, and fair for *all* people, no matter what their race, gender, ethnicity, or nationality happens to be.[17]

In addition to these necessary changes, mankind would also have to completely do away with all of the inner-city ghettos, such as the poor black communities that often feed discouragement, hopelessness, resentment, anger, and aggression, etc. — the demoralizing, underlying symptoms or conditions that readily instigate, fuel, and promote black-on-black crime. And then, they would need to mix people of all the different races, ethnicities, and nationalities all together into the same communities, so that they can all live and enjoy prosperity together, rather than being separated by discriminatory walls and fences — the ugly, divisive elements that impede progress towards racial harmony and success. Also, along with these essential physical changes, another important thing that would be required is that all the different races would have to be taught to cooperate and live together unitedly in peace and harmony.

Another important thing that needs to happen is that blacks and other minorities need to be placed in respectful, responsible, and prominent positions, such as teachers, organizers, and leaders, etc. Not just a selected or token few, so as to try to pacify the masses, like what currently exists; but, instead, *large numbers* of them.

---

[17] In reality, what it will really take to make things fair and just for everyone in the United States, and throughout the entire world, no matter what race, ethnicity, nationality, or gender people happen to be, is not separate, but *one* world government ruling or governing over all people in the world.

Doing this will help to remove or take away the false image and negative stigma that's often associated with blacks, such as them being incapable; or inferior to whites as far as intelligence and other things are concerned. In other words, the image of blacks in general must be changed from a negative one to a positive one. Or to put it or say it ever so bluntly, we (society as a whole) have to completely destroy or kill the "False Image" of the 'Negro' that has been passed down from slavery. But, also, equally important, there is another separate and different image from the erroneous black image of the African American that must also be destroyed, which is the image or false notion that whites are better or superior to blacks and other people of color. This is the only way to effectively improve race relations among all races of people, and to correct and remove the ongoing problems of racial injustices and social inequalities that blacks and other minorities find themselves up against today, and to end racism once and for all time.

All of these things of course are much easier said than done. For it would require, not only a huge undertaking and tremendous efforts, but it would also drastically upset the lives of the rich, powerful, financially affluent and privileged ones. Because in order to equal things out for everyone, they would have to share their space and wealth.

Yes, setting a fair, equal, and just, *balanced* system and arrangement into place would be an important factor for bringing about real change. But, equally important, something else would also be vitally required. And that is a robust educational program would need to be put into place to teach and reshape peoples' minds, hearts, and viewpoints; starting from their youth on up, as to how they view and treat their fellow citizens. In effect, they would need to be *taught* and also *shown* by example on a consistent and daily basis that no race, ethnicity, or nationality is inferior or superior, but rather that they are all equal, and therefore must be highly valued, treated with fairness, dignity, honor, respect, and genuine neighborly love. Some of the ways that this education can be disseminated is through books that are written and geared with this motive in mind, and also through movies, television, the internet, and other forms of social media.

Notice that I said that the end goal is that *all* people must be highly valued and treated with fairness, dignity, honor, love, and respect. Yes, it is how people are *viewed* and *treated* that really counts! Of course, it's one thing to teach or say these things, like some people do, who only want to impress others for personal gain (like some windy, hot air Politian; or a hypocritical religious leader, etc.), but an entirely different thing to truly *act* on what you are saying or teaching—to actually put these things into daily practice in your personal life.

Of course, both taking on and accomplishing all of the positive things mentioned above would not be an easy task, because these things cannot be forced upon anyone. People must come to recognize or see a need in themselves to change, and then willingly work hard at doing it. In other words, people would need strong and proper *motivation* to change—a motivation that stems from a true love of God and one's fellowman.

In addition to being taught racial and social equality, there are also certain damaging bad traits that many people possess that would need to be discouraged or squashed, such as dishonesty, greed, rivalry, etc — disruptive and subversive qualities that work against peace, love, and unity. Unfortunately, removing or suppressing these negative and bad characteristics in people would not be easy, because for many, these things have become so common place or deeply rooted in their mind and heart.[18]

Another reason why it would be important to gain control over, and suppress bad traits such as dishonesty, greed, rivalry, etc., is because even if the problem of racism was totally fixed and cured, there is always the probability that there will be people who will come up with some diabolical plan or way of dividing people for the purpose of exploiting or taking advantage of them for personal

---

[18] As far as the human race is concerned, all people have bad qualities or traits to a certain degree. This is due to everyone being born into sin and imperfection. However, these things can be tamed and suppressed to a large degree if one consciously works on them. On the other hand, the opposite also holds true, and that is if we feed them they will grow.

or financial gain, which is a very good chance it would happen, due to the fallacy and imperfection of man.

With all of the above being said, we can clearly see that it would take enormous reorganization and building efforts to both setup and maintain a balanced system or arrangement of things that would be totally just and fair for all.[19]

Racism — a global issue. Really, when we look at the larger picture of things, we find that racism is not just an American problem. But instead, it is a worldwide pandemic! Because what affects people in one land or area, in effect happens to us all. We may personally think that because we are not a person of color or a minority, or we may happen to be one who currently doesn't seem to be touched by the problem, that it doesn't have anything to do with us personally. But, in reality, it does. The reason why is because we are all closely linked together, in that we are all part of the same worldwide human family, which is the human race. Therefore, racism is a crime, not just against one particular race of people. But rather, it is an immoral crime against all humanity![20]

The root sources of racism are ignorance, hatred, and greed. One example of this is when hate groups from one country target and attack people from another country. Another example is what German Dictator, Adolf Hitler, and his minions did to the Jewish people during the horrific time of The Holocaust (1941-45).

This is just a couple of examples of why the problem of racism has to eventually be addressed and fixed once and for all time, not just on a small scale, such as in the U.S. alone, but on a large scale

---

[19] Although man is limited in what he can do and accomplish, God, the Almighty one who created the entire universe and everything in it is not. For the Bible informs us that he will bring about positive changes for the earth and humankind in the near future. For a list of some of the things that he will do, see the information "Coming, Positive, Future Changes," in Appendix A, on pages 246-247)

[20] As respects humankind, essentially, all of us have the same roots or blood ties, because the entire human race has descended from the first human pair, Adam and Eve. (Genesis 1:26-28)

that encompasses the entire world. A few important reasons why is because it the good, right, and proper thing to do. Another is so that history doesn't repeat itself.

Personal Effects of the False Image

Unfortunately, the "false image," which initially resulted from the intentional slander or character assassination of the African slaves true identity in the past, has had far reaching affects, in that not only has it been passed down from generation to generation, but, also, today, it has spread to affect other people of color too (other minorities), with the black race, overall, sustaining the greatest brunt of the damage.

I too, being born a recipient of this great inhumane travesty, have come to realize that the "false image," along with the resulting established system that was set up to discriminate against people of the black race—the discouraging and destructive *environment*, which I grew up in, and have long lived within ever since, is the root cause or main source of my clinical depression — an illness that progressively grew over an extended period of time, until a final emotional trauma triggered the on-surge of bipolar disorder, as I will explain later in further detail.[21]

Undeniably, the "false image" has disrupted and destroyed many black lives, both past and present. True, as far as personal affects to each and every one goes, it has affected some less or more than it has others. But, overall, the number of casualties, along with the hurt and pain it has caused people of color throughout North American history has been extremely vast and significant.

Today, if the entire black race could and would legally sue the United States Government for restitution, personal injury, or

---

[21] "Environment" meaning: All of the external factors that have a formative influence on a person's physical, mental, emotional, and moral development. To note influence of environment, see the information "Effects of Environment," in Appendix A, on pages 230-237)

impunity damages for the pain and suffering that they have undergone as a direct or indirect result of black slavery, and the "false image" that it created, it would go completely bankrupt. I'm not saying that blacks are entitled to these monies. Nor am I bringing this issue up to provoke an argument or fight. I only convey this in this way or fashion in order to emphasize both the magnitude and seriousness of the problem.

It is important to note at this time, that those who govern the United States today, did not bring about or cause institutional black slavery that occurred in the distant past.[22] But rather, they have inherited the burdensome problems and challenging tasks of trying to pick up the pieces and rectify the ensuing aftermath of the serious issues and problems that slavery caused. However, because some past U.S. Presidents, starting with the very first President, George Washington, were in themselves slave owners that owned plantations, even during the time when they were acting as President and responsible leaders, they are indirectly a big part of the underlying problem of the racism and divisions that exist in America today. For their poor examples and lifestyles promoted and influenced the acceptance and continuance of black slavery in America. It also kept alive the disgraceful, negative, and degrading "false image" of the black race that slavery produced; a distorted, erroneous, hurtful, and damaging image, which has been passed down through time, by means of racial stereotypes and discriminatory practices against the black race, which has contributed to them being victims of modern day era's of segregation, divisions, inequalities, injustices, oppression, and racism. (For further information on this, see "The Foundation of America," in Appendix A, on pages 218-222)

Interestingly, the Churches of Christendom also bear a large brunt of the burden of guilt for slavery and its aftermaths, because

---

[22] I would like to add that although those who govern the United States today are not guilty of intuitional slavery that occurred in the past, they are however guilty and responsible for either implementing laws or allowing laws that were made in the past to continue that favor discrimination against blacks and other minorities.

they idly stood by and said and did nothing to condemn, prevent, or stop this terrible, immoral crime from happening. But instead, they often condoned and supported it.

Concerning the undeniable involvement or role of the church in slavery, former British Prime Minister, Winston Churchill, in the fourth volume of Winston Churchill's History of the English-Speaking Peoples, stated: "Over six hundred and sixty thousand [660,000] slaves were held by ministers of the Gospel and members of the different Protestant Churches. Five thousand Methodist ministers owned two hundred and nineteen thousand [219,000] slaves; six thousand five hundred Baptists owned a hundred and twenty-five thousand [125,000]; one thousand four hundred Episcopalians held eighty-eight thousand [88,000]; and so on. Thus the institution of slavery was not only defended by every argument of self-interest, but many a Southern pulpit championed it as a system ordained by the Creator and sanctified by the Gospel of Christ."

The truth is, history has shown that hypocrisy and religion often goes hand-in-hand, like the false religious leaders (scribes and Pharisees) in ancient Bible times who preached and put forth a showy display of piety (a devout adherence to God or a religion), but in reality their actions were completely out of harmony with their words. Interestingly, Jesus Christ called them blind guides, and hypocrites. (Matthew 23:13-36)

In conclusion, final assessment, and summation of the crux of the matter, in regards to the "false image," along with the discriminatory environment that it created, and the negative and damaging effects that they had on me personally. I believe that they are the primary culprits that ultimately caused my bipolar disorder, as I will now go on to further explain and prove. And to be open and honest with you, it was a very painful and difficult thing for me to have to recall and write about many of the things of my past. I really didn't want to do this. Nevertheless, I realize that it is all part of self awareness, and the healing process. For to keep things bottled up inside can only make matters worse. Often, it is best to open up and talk about it, so that you can get these things off of your chest so to speak, and from that point forward to start the healing and recovery process. Well, with this having been said, and now that all of the background information is in, and the stage is set for the time period, situation, and future environment in which I would eventually be born into and grow up in. Please continue to follow along, as I go on to explain.

Chapter 3

EARLY LIFE AND BEYOND

Although it may be the case for some people, I don't believe that my bipolar disorder is due to genetics, but rather, that it began and developed over an extended period of time, through a series of stages, which were: (1) *bouts of depression,* (2) that gradually and progressively escalated to *chronic depression or mental illness,* (3) which in turn led to an *emotional trauma* that finally triggered *bipolar disorder.*

As I indicated in chapter two, I personally believe that environmental factor and influence played a significantly large role in my developing bipolar disorder, which is a theory that I will now attempt to prove.

First of all, let me start by reiterating that I am a person of mixed-race. I was born in the year 1956, in the city of St. Paul, Minnesota — the child of an interracial marriage, during the time of deep seated racial prejudices, dissention, and segregation in the United States of America, when the African-American Civil Rights

Movement (1954-1968) was in full swing.

My father, Charles Shelton Sr., whom I was proudly named after, was both of African American and Native American decent. And my mother Kathryn was French and Irish (or Caucasian). Interestingly, as a result, from society's standpoint, I was considered "Black" from the moment of birth, although I was mixed or multi-raced, and also fair skinned in complexion.

Because of being born part black, which is something that I am very proud of; unfortunately, I've had to deal with and endure racism all my life, along with the entire black race. However, in regards to my different and unique situation (that of growing up in the fifties, sixties, and seventies, when being mixed-raced and light skinned was rare, particularly in the state of Minnesota where I lived), I believe that for me it was a whole lot worse than it was for the black race in general. The reason being is that I had to deal with discrimination and racism, not from just the white race alone, but also from the black race as well. Because many dark skinned blacks are prejudice towards blacks who are lighter skinned, which often leads to these one's being hated, ostracized, and rejected by them. And because of this, growing up, I often felt like I was sitting all alone in the middle of a fence that was situated in between the two opposing and warring sides, with whites being on one side of the fence, and blacks being on the other.

Another thing that made my plight with racism worse than it was for the black race in general, was that at least they (darker skinned blacks) could identify with one another. And they also had the encouragement and support of one another. I didn't. Because growing up during that racially troubled and divided time in history (1950s-1970s); in the often emotionally reserved and cold state of Minnesota, if you were mulatto or mixed-race, you were an extremely rare and lonely breed. The result was, on the one side, the white race in general viewed and treated me simply as a "Negro," or a "Colored person," one who was part of a weaker race, with inferior intellectual capabilities, etc... in comparison to themselves. And on the other side, the black race customarily rejected and persecuted me for being part white. To them, I was the oddball or freak that stood out like a sore thumb. Subsequently, as a consequence, I for the most part, became a loner early in life. It's not that I preferred it to be that way. It's just that I simply had no other choice. Sure, I had a few friends at times (both white and black), but for the most part, I kept to myself.

What is interesting is that, although the "false image" is a major contributor to my depression; it isn't the only part of the problem. Another significant reason is my being treated as an outcast from people of my own race, along with the fact that I've been forced to sit on the symbolic fence between the white and black races, both of which have failed to open up and fully recognize and accept me for who I am.

Unfortunately, growing up, I'd have to say that the racism I received from both the white and black races was pretty tough on me. And ever since then, I've had to struggle with trying to fit in and find myself in the cold, troubled, and lost world around me.

What is strange is that, when I was growing up as a youth, I was often treated a whole lot worse by the black race, than I was by the white race. Interestingly, I believe that this was due to the notion or teaching that trickled down throughout U.S. history, from the distant past; which was the thought that during the time of black slavery in America, that *"mulattoes"* were used as servants or 'House Negros' in the Master's house, which allegedly was a more favored and less physically demanding position than it was for the darker skinned blacks, who were forced to work as 'Field Negros' in the cotton fields, etc. Apparently, as a result of this difference in treatment, darker skinned blacks developed an aversion or hatred for lighter skinned blacks.[23]

---

[23] A mulatto is a person who has been born from one white and one black parent. In regards to a mulatto living during the time of black slavery in America, the white slave owner or one of his white offspring was the father of the mulatto child. Note: As respects myself, I am not considered a mulatto by the definition of the term, because I have an additional race in me (Native American), along with white and black.

Whatever the reason, the overall racist treatment that I received was a whole lot worse for me, than it was for the average black person in general. Because I was getting it from two sides—from both whites and blacks.

Interestingly, because of my being forced into the position of being at odds with both the white and black races for so long a period of time (throughout my entire life); I think that perhaps this is why I thought that it was both a white man and a black man that entered the bathroom on the day that I was at the hospital, when I was experiencing a panic attack, along with a psychotic episode, which I had referenced earlier in the introduction of this book. Perhaps, in my mind, because of the way that I have been unjustly viewed and treated by them (the white and black races), that they both had become somewhat of an adversary or foe that day — adversaries whom I feared and felt were out to cause or do me harm. Who knows? Whatever the case, it's both curious and amazing how the mind sometimes works.

The False Image Wreaks Havoc!

The "false image" which I defined and spoke about earlier, that has fostered discrimination and racism against the black race, literally has tormented my heart, mind, and soul; not to mention the harmful and lasting effects that it might have had on my siblings or brothers and sisters.

In regards to my family of orientation, I come from a fairly large one. I was born one of nine children. To be exact, I am the sixth one in line from the eldest. The second to the oldest sibling is Caucasian. The rest of us kids are mixed-race.

Although, I have five brothers, they happen to have a different father than me and my three sisters, which makes them biologically our half brothers. But we all have the same mother. And we all at one time or another lived together in the same house.

Oddly, during the time when my siblings and I were growing

up as kids, white people in the community would often stop; frozen in their tracks, and rudely stare at us in public places (at grocery stores, etc.), like we were circus sideshow freaks or something; even though we were somewhat physically attractive people, as far as outward appearances are concerned. The reason they did this is because during that particular time period in history, interracial marriages were rare and few, which resulted in their being only a small handful of mixed raced people in our community; something that they were not used to seeing. Our mother used to get so angry and annoyed with them, that she would stop and fearlessly stare right back at them. And then she would boldly speak up and say to them: "Why don't you take a picture? It'll last longer!"

Sad to say, my fellow siblings and I also suffered a lot of abuse from our black neighbors and school mates too. One of the major reasons why is because they didn't like the fact that we had a white mother. And because of this they would often call us mean and cruel things such as: Uncle Toms, freaks, half & half, yellow bananas, old yeller, and so forth. But little did they know or realize that they were the ones that were really missing out. Because having a Black/Native American father, and growing up in a loving household with a Caucasian mother, and older white brother, was a beautiful, wonderful, and great experience! I wouldn't have exchanged it for the whole world! Because, for one thing, it showed me that all people are equal no matter what their race, nationality, ethnicity, or origin happens to be. And secondly, it also helped to convincingly disprove the blatant and gross lie that has been circulated throughout American history, which is the false notion and teaching that the black race is intellectually inferior to the white race.

Growing Up in a Negative Household

My mother Kathryn grew up in an all female, Catholic orphanage. She was there because her mother tragically died from a massive brain hemorrhage; and her father later suddenly and mysteriously disappeared, and was never to be found. Henceforth, she was awarded to the state of Minnesota, and placed in the

Orphanage. She was only three years old at the time.

Mom lived at the orphanage until she turned eighteen. And then she was free to go. Unfortunately, life at the orphanage wasn't always a good thing for her. Sadly, like a broken, skipping record, she would often tell my brothers and sisters and I, over and over again, nightmare stories about how badly she was treated by the Nuns at the orphanage. The strange thing is, now that I have grown older and I look back at this, to a certain degree (although it wasn't right) I can now understand why the Nuns may have acted the way that they did. No doubt, it was because it was a coldhearted, overly negative, critical, and restricted environment, which was run by impersonal, unaffectionate women that had the practice of suppressing their natural maternal, feminine feelings and emotions.

Later, after leaving the orphanage, and over the course of many years, my mother married several times. And she eventually came to have a total of nine children. That's a lot of kids, especially in respects to most families today, who often, because of modern day practices, traditions, and philosophies; and also because it is much harder to raise children these days; they decide to limit the number of children they have.

In regards to my mother's family of orientation (the family she was born into); she was not an only child. She had five siblings, both brothers and sisters. Strangely, I have to admit that I know little to nothing about them. The reason being is that mom never really talked much about them. However, later in life I got a chance to meet a couple of them.

Prejudice from Within

Oddly and strangely, my mother, although being white, also had to deal with racial prejudice from both the white and black races. Sadly, when she married, her own family even cut her off and disowned her! Apparently, the reason being is because she married into the African American race. Obviously, her family was pretty racist. Because of this, we as her children grew up not knowing our aunts and uncles on our mother's side of the family. The sad thing is, when our mother died from cancer at the age of seventy three, only two of them bothered to come to her funeral. Personally, as it turned out, those were the only two of my mom's siblings that I ever met in my life.

Most assuredly, all of the trying and difficult things that my mother went through in life must have been absolutely devastating to her. I can't even imagine what it would have been like to be so young and have your mother die; and for your father to disappear. And then, in addition to these horrible and heartbreaking things, to be thrown into a cold and impersonal orphanage. And finally, to have your brothers and sisters stripped away from you at an early age, and later to have them disown you. How sad!

In addition to all of the things above, Mom also had to cope and deal with prejudices from people of the black race too, in particular, those who frowned and looked down upon interracial marriage between a white woman and a black man.

Unfortunately, all of the bad experiences that my mother went through in life had a very negative and harmful effect on her, so much so that they ultimately influenced and shaped her into becoming an overly pessimistic and negative person, which is totally understandable. However, despite this, overall I'd have to say that my mother was a very beautiful person by nature. She was also a great mother. Affectionately, she meant the world to me and my siblings! At heart, she was a very kind, generous, and good person; one who dearly loved her children. She was also an immaculately clean and organized housekeeper, as well as an excellent cook. Interestingly, a black woman, named Tassie-May, taught her everything that she knew about cooking. Her fried chicken was to die for!

Our mother could also be extremely gentle, nurturing, and self-sacrificing. One example of this is when I was growing up as a young boy. For some unknown reason, I frequently used to get these painful ear-aches during the late hours of the night. Nevertheless, mom would never get upset with me for disturbing and interrupting her sleep. But instead, she unhesitatingly would quickly rise up; place some drops of appropriate medication in my ear; hold me in her arms; place a hot water bottle (wrapped in a protective cloth) over my ear; and then she would gently rock me in her arms until I fell back to sleep. To this day, I am still very thankful and appreciative to her for her tender, loving care.

Sad to say, however, because of her negative upbringing and bad experiences in life, for the most part, mom was a very negative person. When I was growing up, sometimes it used to drive me nuts. I would think to myself, concerning her often downbeat disposition: *"How in the heck can you be so negative?"* But, now that I have grown older, and I look back at her life, and the many trying and difficult things that she had to deal with and endure, I can better understand why.

Racism's Insidious Nature

Today, the "false image" that portrays the black race and other people of color in such a negative light and inferior way, is so pervasive, saturated, and widespread throughout society, that it has affected and influenced so many people to be racist — even those in Christendom that consider themselves to be Christian. The bizarre thing is many people don't even realize that their thinking and actions have been unduly shaped by it. And if you were to point out to these ones that their viewpoints and actions are racist, they would think that you are highly mistaken, or that you are being overly sensitive. The reason being is because people can so easily be blind to themselves. Often, they don't see themselves for whom or what they truly are. Sure, they may know from the teachings of the Bible that God is impartial, and that he does not approve of racial discrimination in any form. (Acts 10:34, 35) But, nevertheless, because of the strong influence and teaching of the "false image," and the spirit of racism which it has spawned (it being so extensive and far-reaching throughout society), it can be so easy to have this unhealthy, divisive mindset insidiously influence one's thinking and actions — even if it is only to a minimum degree.

What makes racism hard to detect within ourselves is that it can unknowingly or unconsciously be programmed into a person psyche. For example, my mother, who was a Caucasian person, was raised in a predominately white, Catholic orphanage from the time she was three years old — up until she turned eighteen. Now, in that highly protective, sheltered, and enclosed environment you would think that she would be safe and free from the teachings and influence of racism. However, sad to say, she told us (her children) that she was taught by the Nuns there, that black children were little picaninnys.[24]

Unfortunately, this racist teaching and negative viewpoint of blacks that the nuns had went on to influence my mother's thinking to a certain degree.

One day, I remember mom making an offbeat comment about a black and white interracial couple that we were observing in public at a local grocery store. She said, concerning the black man: "Look at him. He thinks that he's better because he has a white woman." At the time I thought to myself: *"Wow... that's a negative and racist remark!"* But not only that, it totally surprised me, especially seeing that it was coming from my mom; a white person who is married to an African American man; and also one that has mixed-race kids herself.

The fact of the matter is, many white people don't see or view people of the black race as being equals. Often, they look down upon them as being less of a person, less intelligent, not as morally upright, less spiritual, not as physically clean, and so forth... in comparison to whites. What's interesting is that even though some may have this thinking or viewpoint, they still don't consciously see or view themselves as being racist.

In truth, though; knowing my mother, I can honestly vouch for her, and say that, in her heart, she was really not a racist person. Overall, she had great admiration for and also a deep respect for

---

[24] A picaninny is a highly offensive and derogatory term that is used for a black child.

African Americans. Also, she loved her husband and her children dearly. However, her thinking to a minimal degree was influenced when she was growing up in the racist environment around her, which caused her to unconsciously make such a senseless statement; that she later regretted and apologized for making.

Negativity's Affect

Growing up in a negative household was very hard on me and my brothers and sisters. As a result, some of us grew up struggling to combat negative thoughts and feelings later in life. Because, unconsciously, negativity was so ingrained in us from early age, onward. It wasn't that my mother deliberately taught us to be critical or negative; it was just that the multitude of bad experiences that she suffered in life ultimately shaped her into becoming the negative person that she became. Personally, I felt sorry for her. But at the same time, I hated and despised the negative outlook and perception of people and things that she often displayed.

On the other hand, despite her often negative nature, I also recall that mom did many positive things to help and encourage others. For example, at a very early age she put me in swimming lessons. I was about seven years old at the time. Later, she enrolled me in summer basketball camps, starting when I was about 11 or 12 years old. Interestingly, I think I was the only one of her children that she did these things for. Now that I reflect back on this, I think it was because she knew my personality or character makeup. And she realized that she had to keep me busy, so as to keep me occupied, and also on the right path, especially with all of the bad influences in the community or neighborhood in which we lived. It's not that I was a bad kid or anything, because I wasn't. Whatever the case, I remember her always saying concerning me: "Chuckie is a deep thinker! That's not good."[25] What mom meant by this, I don't know. All I know is that she wanted the best for

---

[25] My real or legal name is Charles, but my mom, family, and friends called me by my nickname, which was Chuckie.

me, and she took whatever steps or measures necessary to help keep me safe, and also busy, and in good and healthy, productive pursuits.

Influence of an Insightful Father

Unfortunately, my mother and father separated and divorced when I was very young. Nevertheless, my father loved me a lot. He was very proud of me. He even named me after him, which made me a junior. During his scheduled parental visits, he took me everywhere that he went. And he would frequently show me off to his friends, and others.

Sometime later, after my parents' divorced, I went to live with my father for about a year or so. What I remember most about him is that he was a very loving father, and an extremely good provider; so much so, that there wasn't anything that our family was in want or need of. For example, our refrigerator and cupboards were always full and well stocked with various types of foods.

My father was; as you might say, a functioning alcoholic. But he was also a workaholic too. As a matter of fact, he worked two regular jobs throughout his life. At his main job, he worked as "Head Waiter in Charge" for the Burlington Northern Railway Company. His second job was at the St. Paul, Hilton Hotel, where he also worked as a waiter.

Preparation For What Lies Ahead. Being prepared in advance for what lies ahead in life can be very advantageous and helpful to a person. The advanced training and knowledge can not only help to guide and protect one, but it can also toughen them up by giving them valuable insight on how to handle difficult problems and situations if and when they should ever arise.

My father obviously knew from personal experience that as far as life was concerned, I was going to have a tough row to hoe. So from a very early age he tried to toughen me up, so that I would be

BIPOLAR DISORDER A PATIENT'S STORY

better equipped to handle difficult and challenging situations in the future. As a young child, I didn't know what he was actually doing at the time, but later, when I got older, I came to realize or figure it out.

I remember a time when I was sitting alone with Dad's in his parked car. I was about two or three years old at the time. And he turned to me and said: "Let me see your fist." So I showed him my little balled up fist. And then, he asked: "What are you going to do with that?" To be honest with you, I didn't know or understand why or for what purpose he was asking me this. So I didn't say anything in response.

My father then said to me: "Never back down from anybody! If anyone messes with you, or challenges you to a fight, you fight um! Don't you ever back down from anybody!" Then, he asked: "What's your name?"

"Chuck Shelton," I said to him, with my little, quiet and soft tone of voice.

"What's your name?" He repeated.

"Chuck Shelton!" I replied.

"That's right! You are a, Shelton! And Shelton's are special! You remember that," He said.

In response, I shook my head in agreement, and I said: "Okay."

When I reminisce or look back, in regards to my father's training me, I think: *"Wow... that was a lot of pressure to put on a little kid."* But, my father was no dummy. He knew exactly what he was doing. He was trying to prepare and toughen up his young son in advance, to face and deal with the real, cold, hard, and overly aggressive "dog-eat-dog world." But not only that, at that particular time in history, the community where we lived in the city of St. Paul, Minnesota was a poor, ghetto area that was full of violence and a lot of rough characters. Subsequently, under those types of conditions and circumstances a person needs to know how to both deport and protect themselves.

Evidently, what my father taught me made a deep and indelible impression on my mind and heart. The bad thing is, later, as I grew up, I went through life getting in fights! It's not that I initiated or intentionally picked fights with people, for I wasn't that kind of a person. It's just that when I was challenged, I never backed down. Apparently, the reason being is that I felt that I had to fight to defend and uphold family honor. But, most importantly, it was because, if I didn't, I felt that I would be letting my father down; and that of course is something that I tried very hard not to ever do.

Dad's Reputation

My father was a pretty tough character. Not to me or my siblings or family members, but to some outsiders. As a matter of fact, he had a reputation in the community for being a very intimidating dude. Although, I don't remember a time when he was ever mean to anyone in our family or me, or of him ever yelling or raising his voice at us. But, apparently, in public he could be a very loud, boisterous, and scary individual. Consequently, as a result, everyone was afraid of him. Some even went so far as to say, concerning him: "Chuck Shelton is crazy. He'll kill you!"

It's not that dad was mad or insane, or that he had a violent disposition, or was an actual killer or something; it's just that he didn't take any abuse or crap from anybody. Sometimes in life (depending on the area, surroundings, or a particular situation or circumstance that one finds themselves in) a person has to display a hard front, or put forth a good bluff, in order to keep people from pushing them around or taking advantage of them. Whether this was a subterfuge or tactic that my father used, I really don't know. All I know is that, for the most part, people didn't dare to mess with him.[26]

---

[26] Growing up, I use to think that professional boxer Cassius Clay (Muhammad Ali) was crazy because of the way that he acted or the things that he would say or do, especially when he was around or near opponents that he was

Another thing that perhaps intimidated people, with respects to my father, was that they knew that he was a collector of weapons. This was not done for wrong motives, or cynical, or unhealthy reasons, it was simply because dad was a military veteran who served in the U.S. Army; and he liked to collect unique weapons. As a result, over a period of time he accumulated various types of guns, knives, Japanese swords, etc., that he had purchased when he was serving overseas in the military. It's not that he would have ever used these things on anyone, but the image that it projected of him having weapons, perhaps rattled some people.

To give you an example of how my father was respected and feared. One day, when I was young boy, my mother drove and dropped both my younger brother, and myself, off at the local barbershop to get haircuts. We were roughly about eight and four years of age at the time.

Suddenly, a stranger entered the barbershop looking for a job. Quickly approaching the proprietor, whose name was Owen; he proceeded to ask him to hire him as an barber to cut peoples hair.[27]

Owen, who apparently had never seen or met the man before, respectfully said to him: "I'm sorry, but I'm not looking for any help at this time." However, the man refused to take no for an answer.

"Come on, give me a chance!" the Man said.

"No. I'm sorry. But I'm not hiring. Besides, how do I know if you can even cut hair?" Owen replied.

---

scheduled to fight in an upcoming bout... for example when he was to fight Charles "Sony" Liston for the world heavyweight title in 1964. However, it wasn't that Mr. Clay was actually nuts or crazy as Sonny believed him to be. It was just that Cassius tactfully used this fear that Sonny had to psychologically gain the upper hand on him. Interestingly, this feigned disguise worked well for Clay, because he amazingly went on to win the heavyweight title.

[27] The name has been changed.

"I'll prove it to you!" the Man said. And then, turning and pointing directly at me, he said: "I'll cut his hair!"

"Oh no. You don't want to touch his head!" Owen cautioned the man.

"Why not," said the Man.

"Do you know whose son that is?" Owen asked.

"No," the Man replied.

"That's Chuck Shelton's son! And if you touch his head, his dad will kill you!" Owen said.

"Oh yeah, right?" the Man smiled and said, imagining that Owen was just kidding.

Owen now turned, and he looked the man directly in his eyes (as if to get his strict attention). And he said to him with a solemn look on his face, and a tone of sincerity in his voice, saying: "No. I'm serious! He *will* literally kill you!"

After this the man stopped asking Owen for a job. And then, he immediately left the building.

Down to this day and forever, I will always remember that unforgettable day at the barbershop. For dad definitely left quite an impression on many people.

Sad to say, to both my shock and grief, about three years later, in the year 1968, when I was 11 years old, pops passed away from leukemia. He was only 42 years old at the time.

Early Emotional Trauma

One day, when I was about twelve years old, my friends and I were out walking casually through the neighborhood, when all of the sudden, we came upon the body of a dead man lying in the street, next to the curb. It was a black man, who appeared to be in his early to mid forties. He was lying in the gutter. The shockingly thing was that his head was completely severed or cut off, with only just a little bit of skin on one side of his neck holding it on! It was the most horrific sight I had ever seen! Immediately, we ran to our homes (in a small, low-income project housing community), which was located around the corner from where we were, and we told our parents.

After quickly informing our parents about the extremely shocking and horrible sight that we had just witnessed, I don't know why, but for some reason, my friends and I went back to the chilling and gruesome crime scene. Perhaps, it was because we wanted to show them where the body was? Or maybe it was just out of continued curiosity? Or it could have been that we didn't want to be left all alone at home knowing that everyone was leaving to go and see for themselves what had happened? Whatever the case, eventually, there we were once again standing at the terrifying crime scene.

After my friends, and I, and our families approached the dead body, the police eventually arrived at the crime scene. And also a large and growing crowd of concerned and curious people started to assemble and gather around.

Now, for some unexplained reason, the body of the dead man remained uncovered during the entire period of time that we were there. I don't know why, but the police didn't even bother to throw a blanket or sheet or anything over him, to cover the grisly and shocking sight!

I don't remember how long we were standing there at the crime scene, but eventually it started to grow dark. And then, suddenly, a few curious teenage girls, who were traveling together in a small group, showed up.

As the girls began making their way through the large crowd of people, for the purpose of getting a closer look at what it was that we were actually seeing or witnessing; one of the girls, a very pretty girl, with a effervescent smile and lively spirit, who was leading the way, smiled and look at me, and said: "What's going on here?"Apparently, she didn't have a hint or small clue that the body of a dead man was lying stretched out in the street gutter nearby. But, before I or anyone else could say anything to her, she quickly got to and spotted the body. And then, she started frantically screaming and crying out loud, saying: "Daddy! Daddy! Oh no! It's my Daddy!

How shocking and heartbreaking! The poor girl was so traumatized and upset at seeing her dead father, that she literally had to be picked up and carried away from the crime scene. Wow, that's something I will never, ever, forget!

What a horrible and unexpected tragedy! I felt so bad and sorry for the girl!

Personally, because the traumatic scene and images were so graphic and devastating to me, afterwards I couldn't sleep for days!

Unfortunately, back then, in the mid to late 1960s, most minorities and people in the poor communities, like I lived in, didn't seek or get professional mental healthcare, or help for emotional traumas, or clinical depression, etc. Because, either they didn't have healthcare coverage, or it was just too expensive to afford. As a result, if you had psychological issues or problems that should be addressed, it was something that you just had to learn to live and deal with, and try to get through the best way that you could on your own.

Later, upon completing their investigation of the crime scene, the police revealed that they believed that the dead man was a passenger in a moving vehicle; and that he was shot in the neck at close range with a sawed-off shotgun, and then thrown from the vehicle.

A Sad and Memorable Time Period

Up until the year 1967, my brothers and sisters and I attended predominately black schools in St. Paul, Minnesota. But then, in 1967, there was a drastic change. Following the Civil Rights Act of 1964, which ended racial segregation in schools in America, we, along with other black and minority kids, were now being bused to all white suburban schools. The school that my younger sister, and my little brother and I were bused to was called "Como Park Elementary School."

At Como, there were just two minorities in my classroom. Me, and one other black kid, who was darker skinned. The rest of the class consisted of all white kids.

One day, in early April of 1968, while both I and my siblings were in class, my mother unexpectedly arrived and checked us out of school early; although the school day was far from being over. She told us that she came to retrieve us, because Civil Rights Activist and Leader, Martin Luther King Jr., was shot and killed, and that she wanted to get us out of school, and take us home, because she was fearful that riots were about to break-out in the area. Luckily for us, nothing bad or significant ever happened in our hometown area. However, King's death did trigger riots in many U.S. cities.

Because I was only twelve years old at the time, I was not completely up on or aware of everything that was going on in the political world or society. But I remember that this sad and tragic event had a devastating and mournful effect on a lot of people.

Interestingly, although it had seen its good days, for the most part, I remember the 60's as being a very somber and depressing time period, with a lot of bad and tragic events taking place, such as assassinations of very important people taking place. The first was U.S. President, John F. Kennedy, who was assassinated in November of 1963. And then, Human Rights Activist, Malcolm X in February of 1965. Next, Civil Rights Leader, Martin Luther

King Jr., was gunned down in April of 1968. And then, only about two months later, U.S. Senator, Robert F. Kennedy in June of 1968. Most certainly, and for good reasons, you can see why to me and many others, that this was a very bleak, gloomy, and troubling time period; with death and uncertainty lying heavily in the air. In other words, it was almost as though the sun failed to come out and shine.

Early Signs of Stress and Possible Illness

When I was growing up as a teenager, by nature, I was a very good, mild mannered, and clean-cut sort of kid. I didn't drink alcohol. I never used any recreational drugs. I didn't even smoke cigarettes. The reason why I am telling you this in advance, is so that you understand and realize that the experience that I am about to relate to you was not alcohol or drug related.

My experience was this: Late one night, when I was about thirteen years of age, I had a very bizarre and frightening thing happen to me. The situation was, I had gone to bed and promptly had fallen asleep, but then, for some reason, during the night I prematurely woke up. And when I did, I felt all too strange. I felt as though I was about to lose my mind. Not in the way of going mad or crazy, but in a completely different sense.

It's very hard to explain or put into words how I felt, but to me, it was as though my mind was on the verge of slipping away from me, like it was going to fall into an extremely dark and deep chasm or pit; a prisonlike place or condition where there is no chance or way of returning; an unconscious-like, comatose state, place, or condition, where one loses all their mental facilities and ability to function and think normally. In other words, I would be in sort of a vegetative condition or state, without a functioning brain, living in a lonely place or world, where I would not be able to communicate with family and friends. And where they would not be able to communicate or get though to me.

After realizing that I was up and out of bed, and sensing that I was having a problem, my mother quickly rose from sleep, and came to my rescue. Subsequently, what she did is that she held me in her arms; rubbed my head; and calmed my fears by assuring me that everything was going to be alright.

Oddly or strangely; and I know this is going to sound weird, but the only thing that I personally could do to stop my mind from falling or drifting away into the chasm of darkness or oblivion, was that I had to look at and focus my mind and complete attention directly on a fixed object in the room, which at the time happened to be a lighted table lamp (the only light source that was turned on and illuminated the dark room).

Focusing and concentrating with all my might, I struggled and fought to keep my mind from drifting away. For I felt that if I were to let up just a little, I would quickly lose the battle, and then mentally drift away forever. I was extremely frightened and scared, to say the least! Eventually, after calming down, I was finally able to gain control, and bypass the danger zone.

What it was that triggered this strange attack, I don't know? Perhaps it was brought on by the stress of adapting to and living in a new location or surroundings? For we had recently move into to a new house and neighborhood.

Later, my mother took me to a doctor for a physical checkup. But nothing significant turned up. The only thing that the doctor said was that I had an unusual, low pulse rate, which at that time was about 50 beats per minute.

Interestingly, this strange phenomenon that I had experience happened a few times in my life. One of the last times it occurred was when I was about 47 years old. During that particular attack or episode my wife went for a walk with me outside and supported and comforted me (although she didn't completely understand what was happening to me). Luckily, with her comforting help and loving support, I eventually was able to calm down, regain my composure, and was okay.

What it was that triggered these attacks that happened later in my life, I don't know. But one of the things that I vividly recall that usually happened before each attack, is that I was not able to sleep for a long period of time. Strangely, this state of insomnia would last for days; about a week or so, before ending up in an all out attack.

The last time that I experience one of these strange and scary attacks, was on the day that I had my mental breakdown, which I explained and spoke about earlier in my introduction at the beginning of this book. Luckily, for me, it conveniently happened when I was at a hospital, where I could get the immediate medical attention and help that I needed.

Life as a Teenager

As a teenager, I remember being moody and going through bouts of depression at times, although nothing serious. I believe it was just part of being a normal teen. As a result, there would be days when I would sleep a lot, or stay somewhat isolated and locked up in my bedroom. However, this only seemed to make matters worse.

Luckily, the thing that helped to spare me a lot of boredom was my love for basketball. I couldn't get enough of it! I played and practiced all the time, sometimes up to sixteen hours a day, which may seem overly excessive to some people. However, like many youths, it was my ultimate goal to eventually become a professional athlete. But the thing that separated me from others and made me a better ballplayer was my personal drive and willingness to work hard at it.

Dealing with Prejudice from Within

It was a very challenging and difficult thing growing up in a segregated society. But for some people, like myself, it was even worse living in a so called, *desegregated* one (which was a forced situation or social climate that took place in the United States when

I was in my early teens; after the passing of "The Civil Rights Act of 1964"). What made it difficult was, if you were a mixed-race person back then, like myself (having both white and black blood ties); neither side (the white race, nor the black race) wanted to accept you. To me, it was like sitting all alone on a fence in between the two warring and opposing sides. Unfortunately, the effects can leave a person feeling ignored, lonely, lost, and hurt. I once wrote a short poem about it. It's called *"The Invisible Man."* It goes like this:

> There is an invisible man in a crowd,
>
> He is present, though not seen
>
> He cries out to be heard,
>
> But no one hears a single thing!

~

Unfortunately, I grew up during the era when the United States was steep in racial prejudice and segregation, when Civil Rights Activist, Martin Luther King Jr., was leading the African American protest and fight for freedom, equality, and justice for black people — a discouraging, depressing, and tumultuous time, when blacks' were a hated and oppressed people — when Caucasians viewed and treated them as being inferior, especially in regards to intellectual capabilities.

One important thing to remember or note is that during that time period in history, if you were an African American, it really didn't matter what shade of black you were — whether you were dark complexion, brown, or light skinned. All of us were viewed and treated the same by white society. To them, we were all "Negros," or "Colored People." The reason why I bring this up, is because for some reason there are darker skinned blacks that think that lighter skinned blacks, in some way, had it easier than them. They think that we didn't suffer from the same degree of prejudice that they did. Nevertheless, I can truthfully attest to the fact that many of us did, if not even more. I believe one of the reasons why darker skinned blacks felt this way was because they thought that, because "Mulattos" were born part white that they were given special privileges, or were more readily accepted by the white race, than darker skinned blacks were.

Everyone has a right to their own thoughts and opinions of course. However, personally speaking, although I was light skinned, I don't recall ever receiving any special or favored treatment for having white blood ties. The fact is, many white people also viewed and treated me the same as they did darker skinned blacks — which was that of being inferior to whites. And believe me, it was very hard being viewed and treated this way! But also, in addition to this, I had an even greater issue to deal with than the black race in general. The problem was, not only was I being hated and persecuted by whites for being "black," but I was also badly treated by the black race, who regularly belittled, blackballed, and ostracized me for being part white.

Often, while growing up as a young man, I would be minding my own business; not bothering anybody, when all of the sudden, just out of the blue, some blacks would approach me, and in an ugly, sarcastic tone, with a criticizing and taunting type of attitude or disposition, they would say to me: "Whose side are you on?" In other words, they were trying to get me to pick a side. They wanted me to choose between the white race and black race, as to what side I wanted to be on; which was a very bazaar and strange thing for them to ask or put before me — like I actually had a choice in the matter. In response, I would say to them: "I'm not on anybody's side."

How ignorant or stupid to think that I could and would actually make such a ridiculous choice. But, not only this, even if I could, I wouldn't have done it anyways, because, for me to pick or choose a side, would mean that I would either have to deny my mother, who was white, or my father, who was black/native American; and that's something that I would and could never do. Because they are my parents, and my life! I loved them both dearly! They meant the absolute world to me!

In truth, I have always been very proud to be multiracial—to have Black, White, and Native American heritage. I believe that one special benefit of being multiracial, is that it gives a person a greater, overall picture or perspective of life and things. It helps them to be able to view, see, and appreciate situations, things, and people in a much broader way, and from more than one side.

Dark Skin verses Lighter Skin

I know that it's a strange thing to think that darker skinned blacks would be prejudice towards lighter skin blacks. But it's true. Many of them hate mixed-raced people who are African American, but have white ancestry or blood. It's as though they blame or hold these ones directly responsible for the inhumane crimes and bigoted actions of the godless slave owners who presided over their ancestors that were slaves in past, centuries ago—something that today's "mulattos" had absolutely nothing to do with![28]

One thing in particular that I think has insidiously and strongly served to influence and shape dark skinned blacks prejudices towards lighter skinned blacks, is a story or tale that has been circulated and passed down through time, concerning how slaves were treated during slavery.

I'm not sure when the teaching first manifested itself, but according to rumors or trickledown stories, it's been taught that during slavery light skinned blacks, "mulattos" were given a more favorable position or job, which was that of working as "House Negros" (apparently, because they were the bastard children or offspring of the slave owners); a position which spared them the hard and painful life of working as field hands in the plantation fields; something that black slaves who were not mixed breed were forced to work.

---

[28] Not all blacks who are darker in complexion are prejudice towards lighter skinned blacks. However, from personal experience, this is what I've experienced in general from a big percentage of them. Also, to add insult to injury, if you happen to be well educated, some of them hate you even more. Because according to them, they say: "You're trying to be white!"

I don't know whether the story was true or not, but if it was, when you think about it, if those mixed breeds or mulattos lives were so much better and privileged as was thought, that is, in comparison to the regular field hands, then why did former slave, Fredrick Douglass (who later became known as the Father of the Civil Rights Movement); a person who was mulatto himself, (who was believed to have been the bastard offspring of his slave owner); beat his master with a whip, and then escape to freedom? If being a "mulatto" offered that much better of a life for him as a slave, then why did he highly yearn for his own liberation and freedom, and then eventually flee from captivity? And after having received his freedom, why did he later stanchly fight endlessly for the freedom of other slaves, which included mulattos? Obviously, it was because the effects of slavery was the same for him as it was for all other slaves, no matter how dark or light skinned their complexion happened to be.

The truth is, a slave was a slave, no matter what position, job, or tasks he or she was given to perform. And just like their fellow darker skinned slaves, lighter skinned blacks were also subject to the cruel effects of slavery. They too were denied the rights of education, equality, and freedom!

Another important point to consider is that today's "mulattos" are not the direct offspring of white slave owners that lived in the past, who often raped their slave women; but rather, they are children of modern day interracial marriages and relationships. So why be jealous of these and hate them for something that they had absolutely nothing to do with.

Ironically, in regards to the time period when I was growing up; as it turned out, blacks were fighting for equality in a white world, while I was looking for or more concerned with receiving equal treatment from both sides; the white and black races. For not only was I facing prejudice from the white race for being a minority, but I also had to deal with being rejected and ostracized by the black race for being part white.

Fortunately for me, my mother — God bless her soul — who

lived to be 73 years old, was the only one that held things together for me in a racially divided and troubled world. Her love to me was the only sure thing that made perfect sense to me. She was my "Rock of Gibraltar," my "Bright Shining Star." Unfortunately, when she died, it was a terrible and tragic blow to me, so much so, that afterwards I lapsed into a deep depression, which lasted for about seven years or so.

A Hater of Injustice

Personally, I have always had a strong intolerance for and hatred of injustice. The reason being is that I simply do not like to see people being treated badly or unfairly. It doesn't matter what age, race, ethnicity, nationality, origin, or gender they happen to be. For example, while I was attending grade school in the 8th grade, I observed that the black students in class were being treated badly by the teacher, who was a Caucasian woman. For some reason, she always seemed to single them out and yell at them for one thing or another. Why, I don't know? All I remember is that often the black kids would not be paying attention to what was being taught in class. Instead, they would be talking and joking around amongst themselves.

By nature, I was a pretty quiet kid. And also a fairly good student, that usually did what I was told. And I got good grades. So the teacher never really singled me out or picked on me. But when I observed how the black students were being singled out and treated, I felt bad for them, and so I decided to cast in my lot with them so to speak. The action that I took had nothing to do with peer pressure. I guess I just felt sorry for them. So in response and protest of the matter or issue, what I proceeded to do, was I stopped performing academically for the teacher.

Eventually, as time went by, my recent and sudden lack of production in class worried and puzzled my teacher. She was very concerned as to why my grades had dropped, and why I was no longer as productive of a student as I was in the past. So one day, she privately pulled me aside, and she said to me: "Chuck, your grades have dropped significantly. What's the matter? Is there something wrong?" In response, I kept silent. She continued, saying: "I talked to Mr. Magettie (the previous teacher that I had the year prior to her), and he told me that you got A's and B's in his class.[29] So why aren't you performing for me?" Again, I just kept silent. In the end, she never did quite figure it out. All I know is that she was frustrated that I had quit on her. And that's how I wanted her to feel. I guess this was my way of getting even or back at her for being unjust in her treatment of the black students.

Now, that I am older and wiser; when I look back at the past, I realize that it was a very stupid and foolish thing for me to have reacted this way towards my teacher, for although I did it to be supportive of my peers and to frustrate her, in the long run I was the only one who wound up being hurt, both academically and emotionally. For I had allowed that negative situation to create in me a bad spirit or self destructive attitude, one that ended up influencing and shaping my character to a certain degree, as well as my future viewpoint and outlook about certain things or particular aspects of life.

Pressures of Being a Black Male

When I was about 9 or 10 years old my mother remarried. My new stepfather, Franklin, was an African American man.[30] Unfortunately, later, when I was 18 years old, he and mom separated and divorced. In total they were together for about thirteen years; five of these were before they got married.

When I was about five or six years old, Franklin was an out of work dry cleaner, who worked at a local dry cleaning business. It wasn't that he was lazy or anything. He was just laid off from work.

Unexpectedly, one day, my biological father, Charles Shelton

---

[29] The name has been changed.
[30] The name has been changed. Also, I call Franklin my stepfather, although I was never officially adopted by him.

Sr., stopped by our residence, and he said to Franklin: "Come on Franklin, I'm going to get you a Job. You're going to take good care of my kids!" (The children that were paternally his, which were my three sisters and me). This made a good and big impression on me, because I could see that my dad loved us, and that he wanted the best for us kids.

By nature, my father was a hard worker and good provider, who held down two jobs at the same time, for many years — up until he died, he worked for both the Burlington Northern Railway Company, and also the Hilton Hotel, in downtown St. Paul. At both jobs, he served as "Head Waiter in Charge."

Later that day, to me and my family's joy and surprise, when Franklin returned home, he now had two jobs! One job, was working for the Burlington Northern Railway Company, and the other working at the Hilton Hotel. Apparently, thanks to my father's good name and recommendations, he was hired right on the spot, at both places!

I both loved and respected my stepfather Franklin, and I appreciated what he did for our family financially. He had a big responsibility, because he had to provide for a wife, and many kids, seven of which were his step kids (although, he never did legally adopt any of us). Nonetheless, like clockwork and on a regular basis he would voluntarily hand over his paycheck to my mother, so that she could take care of the household and financial matters. It wasn't that he was incapable of handling these things himself, for he was a pretty smart guy. It's just that he was generous like that.

One thing that I wish is that I could have gotten to know him better. A couple of things that made this difficult at times is that by nature I was an both an introvert and quiet kid; and he was hard to open up and communicate with, at least as far as I was concerned. One reason for this may have been, that for some unexplained reason, during that particular time period in history, adults just didn't communicate with kids the way that we as parents and grandparents do today. Back then, in the past, kids had their separate place in the family and society. For it was a commonly held practice and belief that "kids are only to be seen, and not heard." As a result, this led to many youths growing up feeling ignored, unappreciated, and unloved.

Another possible reason why it may have been difficult for us to get to know each other better is that, like my paternal father, Franklin too was a functioning alcoholic, who was dealing with his own personal problems and issues. Now, I don't condone alcoholism, but I can totally understand why it would be so easy for one to become an alcoholic, especially when you're a black male living in a discriminatory society that views and treats you as being inferior; or one that robs you of your self-respect, dignity, and manhood — something that was the norm for black men living during that difficult time period.

Unfortunately, Franklin died some years back, but the good thing is that I have a great relationship with his surviving son (the only offspring that he fathered by our mother); my little brother, whom I truly love, appreciate, and enjoy, along with the rest of my beautiful brothers and sisters!

High School

When I was a teenager, the high school that I attended was named, "Mechanic Arts," which was located in St. Paul, Minnesota, close to the state capital building. No, it wasn't an automotive repair school, as the name may seem to suggest. It was just a regular, liberal arts high school for boys and girls. Why it was called Mechanic Arts, I don't know.

Although, I was a pretty smart kid, who usually did fairly well in school as far as grades were concerned, I rarely ever truly applied myself academically to any subject. For the most part, I only did what I had to, just to squeeze by, which usually landed me a "B," and an occasional "A" here and there. However, during my 10th and 11th grade years, a girl named Ellie, inspired me to work hard in math class (geometry and trigonometry) to get "A's," something which I managed to achieve. Ellie was really smart. But she was also pretty cute too!

In addition to Ellie's encouragement and positive influence, there's only one other time that I can think of when a subject at school really sparked my interest, and that was the subject of architectural drafting and design. I fell in love with it! In fact, I couldn't get enough of it![31]

One day, when I was in the 9th grade, I enthusiastically said to my architectural drawing teacher: "Teacher, I really like drafting. Teach me more!" He replied: "I'm sorry Chuck, but I've already taught you everything that I know! If you want to learn more, you will need to enroll in a vocational school for architectural drafting and design after you graduate from high school." Sad to say, after hearing this, it left me feeling very disappointed. Because, at the time, three to four years down the road to a young kid my age, seemed like too long of a time to wait. So in the course of time, as the days and months passed, I forgot about it. And I moved on to pursuing a completely different career goal, which was to become a professional athlete.

High School Sports

I was a very successful high school athlete. As a senior I was awarded All City, All State, and All American basketball honors. As it turned out, a couple of these awards in particular were unique and exceptionable individual accomplishments, in that no one in the entire history of Mechanic Arts High School Basketball had ever achieved All State and All American honors. A few athletes prior to me had achieved All City basketball status, but that was it. Interestingly, during my senior season of basketball, one of the local newspaper sports reporter's gave me the nickname "Mr. Cool." I'm not sure why he named me this. But I think it was because of my level headedness and composure on the basketball court during clutch and pressure situations. Whatever the reason,

---

[31] The Name has been changed.

the name stuck with me. But even more rewarding than any personal accolades or individual athletic honors, was the satisfaction and reward of playing on a winning team!

In my final season, and senior year in 1974, as a team captain, I was able to help lead my high school basketball team to an undefeated 16-0 regular conference season, which was an amazing feat, seeing that this had never been achieved before in my school's entire basketball history! That year our basketball team even won the Twin City's Championship Game against the then, undefeated, Minneapolis powerhouse, Washburn High School (who entered the game with a 17-0 record and No. 2 rating amongst the states large schools); a game in which I scored 32 points. This was twice as many points than anyone else scored on either team. But we also beat them convincingly, by 16 points, and the game wasn't even that close.[32]

In an earlier conference matchup game against St. Paul, Johnson High School, I scored 39 points (a season high). This was pretty good considering that I had only played three out of the four regulated quarters.[33]

I loved playing basketball. It had become the love of my life, ever since I began playing it at the very young age of about eleven or twelve. And now, being older and in high school, all of the hard work that I had put in practicing over many years was beginning to pay off.

Coveted School Blanket

At Mechanic Arts, there was an annual school tradition at the end of each school year. The tradition was that they awarded the year's top athlete for his or her athletic achievements that they

---

[32] The Twin Cities Basketball Game was an annual event in which the best Minneapolis school competed in a game against the best St. Paul school.

[33] In 1974 High School Sports, basketball games consisted of four separate quarters or time periods. Each quarter or playing period was eight minutes long, which made for a total playing time of 32 minutes per game.

obtained during the year. The school did this by given out a very special award, which was a highly coveted, special, school blanket. The interesting thing is that it was awarded to only one individual, per school year.

The school blanket had the school colors, also its name, the year, and the name of the winning athlete monogrammed on it, and so forth. It was a pretty big deal! Apparently, the selected recipient of the award was decided upon by the school's principle, and other faculty members.

Because of my individual athletic honors and achievements, and our basketball's team's overall success in 1974, it was common knowledge throughout the school that I was a guaranteed, shoo-in to receive the school blanket award that year. I vividly recall the day when the winner of the award was to be named. It was a big event that was scheduled to be held in the school's large auditorium. My mom was even in attendance that day to witness me receiving the award. But, unfortunately, to the absolute shock and dismay of her and everyone else there, when it came down to announcing the winner, the award went to someone else instead. As it turned out, it was given to a person whom we never would have imagined would even have a chance to win. As a matter of fact, his only affiliation with school sports was that he played on the school's baseball team, which was a weak team that didn't even have a winning season. Sure, he was a nice kid, but he wasn't even a good athlete. What's even stranger or more puzzling is that he literally served as the water-boy on our A-squad basketball team! Truly, it was totally undeserving for him to have been honored and awarded with the distinguished, school blanket, athletic award.

Following the award ceremony, my mother and I walked down to the school's principal office, where she gave him, and a few of the other faculty members that were present (people who were instrumental in choosing the winner of the best athlete award) a piece of her mind.

In trying to save face, the school's principal offered a pretty lame or weak excuse, saying: "Chuck only played one sport, and that's why he didn't receive the award." But, I immediately corrected him. I reminded him that I also ran on the cross-country team during both my junior and senior years at school. And, as a matter of fact, when competing in my very first cross-country contest or meet (when I was in the 11th grade), I shattered our school's record; running faster than anyone in Mechanic Arts High School's entire school history![34]

Still trying to save face, the principal offered another lame excuse. He said: "Chuck never served on the student council." In response, my mom said to him: "What does being on the student council have to do with a sports award?" He had no answer! And then, my mom said to him, and the others that were present: "The reason way you didn't give my son the school blanket award is because you people are prejudice! And after all that my son did for you and this school. How pathetic!" Afterwards, she and I turned and left.

To tell you the truth, it really hurt me that I was passed over for receiving the school's top athletic achievement award. Afterwards, when I got home, I went for a two mile jog. And, along the way, I broke down and cried. I guess it was because I had worked my butt off for many years to be the best basketball player that I could be; in particular, putting in many long hours of practice in the summer, during school breaks. But also, I was a very good and skilled ballplayer that was good enough to have been a starter and team captain on any school team. As a matter of fact, according to a St. Paul, Pioneer Press sports columnist Don Riley, he wrote: "Shelton's the best floor general I've seen since Dick Kaess at Washington in 1942. Also, in the Minneapolis Star and Tribune newspaper, I was named to the first squad, Minneapolis, All Star Basketball Team, which also included some basketball greats that became professional athletes, such as Mark Olberding from Melrose, Minnesota who became a professional NBA basketball

---

[34] The sport of High School Cross-country is a footrace in which teams and individuals compete and run for a distance of 3 miles (4.8 km) over an open-air, natural terrain course.

player, and Jack Morris from Highland Park, Minnesota who became a professional baseball player (pitcher), and was later inducted into the National Baseball Hall of Fame. Interestingly, my high school basketball team beat Jack Morris' (who was also a phenomenal basketball player) basketball team in my senior year. Jack's basketball team came in second place in that 1973-74 city conference season, with a 14-2 record. They suffered only two defeats that year. The only team that they lost to was us, Mechanic Arts, who beat them twice.

In addition to working hard at basketball, in the summer of 1973, right before beginning my senior year, I had even turned down a full sports scholarship that I was offered to attend Cretin-Derham Hall High School, which is a very wealthy, prestigious, and private school. I told a basketball scout who tried to recruit me, that I was very thankful for the generous offer, but that I preferred to finish my high school basketball career at my father's Alma mater, which was Mechanic Arts High School. But also, more importantly, in my mind I was thoroughly determined to use my athletic ability and talent to help Mechanic Arts go undefeated in conference play (something that had never been achieved before in the school's entire history); that is until my team and I was able to finally accomplishment this amazing feat in my senior year of 1974, by achieving a perfect 16-0 record.

In conclusion, because of all of the hard work and individual sacrifices that I made, you can see why I was so disappointed that I did not receive the school's top athletic achievement award — the coveted, School Blanket. But the thing that hurt me the most, was that my school's principle and its faculty members failed to truly appreciate what I had did and sacrificed for them; the school's athletic program; and its overall success.

Chapter 4

DEPRESSION AND

THE WORK ENVIRONMENT

At the young age of twenty two, I married a beautiful Latino woman. This was the happiest day of my life, for as it turned out she is my perfect soul-mate. To tell you the truth, the first time that I saw her, it was love at first sight. During that time I thought to myself: *"Wow... that's the girl I'm going to marry!"* But then, of course, I had to later convince her of that, which she finally accepted. Lucky for me!

Although being happily married, not all was rosy though. It's not that I was unhappy or dissatisfied with my wife or anything in particular. Because I love and cherish her dearly! And she brings me a lot of joy and happiness. The problem was, because of my upbringing, with the often negative outlook, and influence of my mother, along with the negative "false image" that is so ingrained in society that I had to daily cope and deal with. I often struggled to combat negative thoughts and emotions.

Generally speaking, for the most part, I was a very happy-go-lucky sort of person with an optimist outlook. As a matter of fact, I remember that there were many days when my heart actually leaped with joy! However, on the other hand, there were also times or periods when I was moody or crabby—times when I felt like I was down in the dumps and I just couldn't pull myself out. And, believe me, I hated myself for being this way.

By nature, my wife is a wonderful and beautiful person. She has such a positive and healthy outlook on things, and also a natural love for people. One of the outstanding things about her is that she always gives other people the benefit of the doubt. And she always looks for the good in them, rather than the bad. Unlike her, I was often highly suspicious and skeptical of people, and afraid that I was going to get hurt by them, because for the most part, this is what I have experienced in life.

I felt so bad for my wife for having to deal with and put up with my frequent bouts of crabbiness and downcast moods. I desired so much to be more like her—more upbeat and positive. Often, I would say to her: "You're a much better person that I am! I wish that I was more like you!"

Now that I have grown older, I'm beginning to realize that having a love for people is an important factor or key to having a healthier outlook and more joyful life. But also, I'm coming to realize that I have become a lot like my mother, in that I have allowed the many bad experiences that I have gone through in life, to mold or shape me into being the miserable man that I have become.

It is so easy to allow our minds to dwell on the bad or negative things in life, rather than fight against it — to be swept along by a stream of unhealthy thinking and habits that we have developed over time; an ever raging current that can lead us into the sea of darkness and despair. Personally, for me, although the task seemed insurmountable, I was determined to change for the better. However, at that particular time in my life, little did I realize that I was fighting against a powerful, unrelenting enemy—Depression!

Work and Depression

In April of 1979, I started work as a meter reader, working for the local electric company. I was twenty three years old at the time. It actually took me two months to get hired, but after a lot of trying and persistence it eventually paid off, and I finally got the job.

The location where I was hired to work was out at one of the electric company's suburban offices in Brooklyn Center, located in the northern metropolitan area of Minneapolis, Minnesota. At the time, there were only two minority meter readers working there, which was me, and another African American man, who was darker skinned.

After being hired, about eight months later I was transferred within the company to a different location; another suburban office, located in city of Edina, in the southern metro area of Minneapolis, where I happened to be the only person of color.

Personally, I thought that the job of reading meters was great, primarily because it was so easy! Sure, it involved a lot of walking. However, because I was an athlete and always in tiptop physical condition, it made it a breeze. But, there was one thing that made the job very challenging at times, and that was the dread of having to face and deal with dogs. Sometimes the situation was downright unnerving and scary, such as when you're being chased by a big German Sheppard or Doberman Pincher, and their nipping at your heals!

After working as a meter reading for a while, I quickly came to realize that the dogs weren't the only problem associated with the job. There were also some difficult customers too that I had to cope and deal with, such as people who would deliberately let their dogs out on you! Sometimes, I would think that the customer's dispositions were worse than their dogs!

In order to protect meter readers from overly aggressive and attacking dogs, and to eliminate or reduce the number of dog bites, our company conveniently supplied us with mace or pepper spray. And because I was highly fearful of canines, I didn't hesitate to both carry and use it when threatened.

One day, while I was out reading meters, as I walked around the corner of a house, a large dog that had just been given a bath, and was being brushed and groomed by its owner; suddenly broke away from her, and it charged at me. In response, I panicked! Quickly pulling out my pepper spray, I literally sprayed it from the top of its head to the tip of its tail. In response, the owner said to me: "Hey! I just gave him a bath!"

"I'm sorry, but your dog startled and frightened me!" I replied.

"Will that spray hurt him?" She asked.

"No. It's just harmless pepper spray," I said. Afterwards, I thoroughly apologized to the lady for spraying her dog. I informed her that I didn't do it intentionally. But, because of being completely startled… it was due to quick reflex response. She said "Ok." The unfortunate thing is, when I left, she had to give her dog another bath all over again, because the pepper spray that I spayed on him was a vivid, bright orange color, and his fur was a light shaded tan. Oops!

Good Work Ethics

As a meter reader, I was a very hard worker, one who, for the most part, always completed his daily work assignments (meter reading routes).

Initially, after being hired as a meter reader, I, like all new employees, was placed on a six month probationary period. And I was informed by the company that after the completion of that time period, if I had proven to be a good worker, that they would hire me on as a permanent, fulltime employee. Fortunately, in my case, as it turned out, I didn't have to wait the full six months; for my job hired me on permanent at the beginning of my fifth work month. The reason why, Management told me, was that because I was such a good and hard worker that they didn't want to lose me. And so they decided, in my case, to forgo the six month probationary period and make me a permanent employee earlier. This was good news to both me and my wife, because now I would get a substantial pay raise. And also full medical benefits for the entire family, which we didn't have prior to this time.

I loved reading meters, because it was both fun and easy. When I first got hired I couldn't believe that a company would actually pay a person for doing such a physically and mentally easy job. Also, the pay was pretty good too. However, I soon learned that the job was more difficult than it actually seemed or was in the beginning.

Because I was hired in the early spring, when the weather happened to be pretty nice, and there was no snow on the ground (which during that particular time in the snowy and cold state of Minnesota is not always the case), I didn't see the job for all that it really entailed. Later, however, I got a rude awakening when the hot days of summer came, and also when old man winter arrived during the following winter season. For both Minnesota summers and winters can be pretty brutal. The fact is, Minnesota can have extremely hot summers, and also frigid cold winters with heavy snowfall accumulations. Often, the snow can get so deep, that your body is buried up to your waist! Nevertheless, despite these physically demanding and challenging situations, it barely slowed me down on the job, because I was both young and in great physical condition.

I was a runner, who literally ran through my meter reading routes (something that often amused and amazed many of my customers). And on a regular basis, except for certain inclement weather conditions, which I will explain later, I would always complete my daily work assignment, no matter how long or difficult my routes happened to be.

Nowadays, during the timeframe and difficult period that we now live in, with all of the troubles, scares, and problems in the world, I don't think a meter reader could actually get away with running his routes like I did in the past. Today, with people being on edge due to increased crime, violence, and terrorism, etc., and with heightened security everywhere, he'd probably get shot!

On average, I would estimate that the total walking distance of each, separate meter reading route, was about ten miles long. However, some were shorter, and others were longer, depending on the particular area being worked. Interestingly, I was the only meter reader that consistently finished his routes day after day. The rest of the employees would often bring back unfinished work. As a result, my fellow meter readers would often say to me: "Slowdown! You're making us look bad!" One day, one of them even wanted to physically fight me, because I had finished one of his routes that he had never completed before. Luckily, for him, I had recently become a Christian, trying hard to live by the teachings of the Bible, otherwise, I might have taken him up on it. In an effort to maintain peace, I told him that it wasn't anything personal, but that I was only working hard to get the job done, so that I could go home. Unfortunately, after this, he regularly avoided me, and never bothered to talk to me again.

One of the many great benefits of the meter reading job was that it had field release. This meant that if you finished your route early, that you could go straight home afterwards, and not have to return to the office until the following day. This was the case, no matter what time you got done. If your route only took you three hours to read, then you were free to go home. And the beautiful thing was that you still got paid for a full eight hour workday. I loved it! It was great!

Our regular, daily start time for work was 8:00 am. And on average, it would take me only about three hours each day to finish a complete route. And often, I would get done even earlier than this. On average, on a daily basis, I would get home from work no later than about 12:00 pm. It was like having a high paying, part-time job, along with full medical benefits. Yep, it was an awesome arraignment! Or as some would say, "It was a piece of cake!"

One of my younger brothers told me that I didn't know how lucky I was to have the best job in the world! He said, one highly favorable and desirable thing that makes my job so great is because I don't have to deal with the politics and problems that are often associated with working together with other people, such as in an enclosed office space or factory setting. I totally agreed with him, because all I had to do each morning was to report to my job; pick up my route for the day; and then leave and be on my own. It was like being my own boss. I didn't have to deal with or report to anyone (except for at the beginning of each workday when I had to pick up my route), and neither did I have to worry about being micromanaged or having someone constantly looking over my shoulder. I was free to work at my own leisure and pace. And believe me, I worked hard! But also, the daily exercise that I got, along with the fresh air, helped to reduce the daily stresses of life, which was good for my overall health.

Accepting the Bad Along with the Good

Although meter reading was a great job, not all was wonderful or glorious. Because when you're working as a lowly meter reader, you have to put up with being negatively stereotyped. The fact is, most people think the reason why a person reads meters is because they are uneducated or incapable of doing anything else. True, in comparison to some other types of employment, it may not have been the most mentally challenging or prestigious job. However, the great benefits that it offered far outweighed the low-grade image that it presented. Interestingly, my own mother even said to me: "Chuck, you need to get a different and better job. You're capable of much better things! You would make me so proud, if you would become a police officer!"

I told her that I was perfectly happy with my current job, and that the life of a policeman was not for me. For one thing, I didn't want to be put in the compromising position of having to kill anybody. And I definitely didn't want anyone shooting at me. But, not only that, the meter reading job was a much better job in so many ways! It was like my brother said "The best job in the world!"

In total, I worked or read meters for 22 years. And during that time I occasionally suffered from bouts of depression, especially during the dark, cloudy, and cold winter months when the sun rarely shines in the State of Minnesota. But, one vital thing that I think helped and sustained me during this glooming time, was the daily exercise and fresh air that I was getting. Another thing that helped was that I played a lot of basketball. And I also spent a lot of time working out at health clubs.

Exercising and lifting weights was a big part of my life. I think it was in my blood, because I had been involved in these things from a very early age. But also, personally, I've always felt that having good overall conditioning and strong legs were necessary requirements for my job. For it made it a whole lot easier. Because of this I made sure that I always stayed in top physical condition. And because my legs were my "Bread & Butter" so to speak, I especially worked hard to keep them strong. And they were. I could easily hack squat over a thousand pounds; completing ten sets of 10 to 15 repetitions!

Coping with Prejudice on the Job

Although, I had a job where I didn't have to directly work with and around people; I still had to have contact with them in some fashion or form every day, even if it was to a limited degree.

One day, while I was out reading meters at a new housing construction site, located in the northern suburbs of a white community, where a lot of new homes where being built, I happened to run past a construction crew (who were all Caucasian men); that were building a house directly across the street from where I was working.

Upon seeing me, one of the construction workers shouted out a wisecrack or dig that was directed at me.[35] In a loud voice he said:

"Look at that Nigger go! He sure does want him a job!" And then, he and his fellow coworkers busted out in laughter. In response, I quickly turned and looked at them. And although I was both angry and hurt by what the man said, and how I was being ridiculed, I just turned back around and kept on running and reading meters.

~

Another day when I was working, I came very close to being bitten by a dog. What happened was, I was running across the front yard of someone's house, when all of the sudden a large dog came flying around the corner of the house, charging right at me. In quick response, I leaped high into the air, clear over his head. Also, simultaneously (at the same time that I jumped), I quickly grabbed my can of pepper spray that was attached to my shirt pocket, and I sprayed the dog with it, from the crown of his head to the tip of his tail, as he was passing underneath my legs.

Luckily, after I landed back down on the ground, the dog kept his distance from me; although, he was still aggressively looking for an opening to get at me. And then, I heard and saw the dog's owner, who was a Caucasian man. He was standing in the front yard, at the south or opposite end of the house, with a big smirk on his face. Next, boldly and frankly speaking out, the man said to me, as I'm continuing to fight off his attacking dog: "Oh, don't worry; he [his dog] doesn't like Nigger meat!" In response, I looked at the man with a disgusted and repulsive look on my face. And even though I was really angry with him for making such a racist remark, I just shrugged it off, and kept moving on, without even bothering to read his meter, which was located in his backyard.

~

At another time, in the year 1980, while my wife, her sister, and I were vacationing in St. Petersburg, Florida, I happened to be standing outside of a drugstore that was located within a small strip mall. The reason I was there, was that I was browsing through some postcards at a sidewalk sale that they were having, while my

---

[35] A dig is a cutting, sarcastic remark.

wife and her sister were next door washing clothes at a self-service Laundromat.

Like most days in Florida, it happened to be a nice and sunny day. But then, all of the sudden, the weather took a turn for the worse, as dark and heavy rainclouds began to quickly roll in, and loud thunderous noises began occurring in the sky overhead. And then, suddenly, I heard a loud voice talking. It was coming from a man who was standing next to his car that was parked nearby. Also, he had a couple of males with him. From the looks of it, they appeared to be his friends.

Shouting out something, in reference to me, the man said to his friends: "I can't believe a Nigger would still be standing around during a thunderstorm!" And then, he and his friends began laughing their foolhardy heads off at me.

I have to admit that this nasty racist remark made me very angry at the time. And it took a lot of self-control for me to hold myself back. Nevertheless, I just kept silent, and I let it go. Afterwards, I left and joined up with my wife and her sister in the Laundromat.[36]

Manifesting Goodness In
The Face of Adversity

When I worked as a meter reader, I was always courteous and kind to the customers, no matter how cranky or rude some of them could get. One day, as I both knocked and rang the doorbell at a house that was located within a very affluent and rich white community. A woman (who was Caucasian) came to the door and chewed my head off. With a loud and angry tone, she said: "Why are you both knocking and ringing at my door!" Apparently, she thought that this was excessive or overkill. In response, I sincerely apologized to her, saying: "I'm sorry Ma'am, but this is the direct

---

[36] All of the bad experiences involving racial issues that are mentioned above are just a few of the bad experiences that I had in life. There are many more.

instruction and training that I received from my boss. He told me and my fellow coworkers to both *ring* and *knock* at houses that have electric meters in their basement. This way the house owner is sure to hear you, and let you in."

After explaining myself to the woman, she let me in her house and I read her meter, which was located in her basement. And after I was finished, on my way out the door, I made it a point to apologize a second time. Interestingly, a few days later, my boss handed me a written letter to read. It was from the perturbed lady. The letter was addressed to my employer. In a nutshell it said that they are lucky to have such a nice and respectful young man like me working for them.

~

On another occasion, a Caucasian man who had been a very successful salesman for a large percentage of his life, but was now retired, informed me that he had mailed a letter to my company about me. He said that in the contents of the letter he informed my company that I had been reading his meter on a monthly basis for quite some time. He said that personally he had worked as a salesman for over 30 years, and that during all that time never had he ever come across a person like me before. He said that I have wonderful qualities and capabilities. And that I would make an amazing salesman. He told my company that they would do well if they were to invest money in me. In response, I thanked the customer for the wonderful complement and all that he did for me, and then I left.

Several days later, my boss pulled me aside and talked to me privately. And he showed me the impressive letter that the retired salesman had sent, which he had recently received from upper management. Afterwards, he said to me in a tepid and nonchalant manner: "I thought that you might want to see this. I'll put it in your personal file, and keep it there." I thought to myself: *"Wow, here it is that upper management received a glowing letter of complement and recommendation from a highly experienced and successful businessman, concerning me, and they're not even going to do anything about it... to use and take advantage of my youth, abilities, and talents.*" Upon observing their lackluster response and unappreciative attitude, it made me feel sort of sad, but at the same time it wasn't totally unexpected, seeing that minorities aren't always valued and appreciated the way they should be, at least not in certain areas or things in life.

The following month, when I returned to read the retired salesman's meter again, he proudly and enthusiastically asked me if my company had received his letter. I said to him: "Yes." However, because I was too embarrassed to tell him the truth about what had really happened; and I didn't want to discourage him or hurt his feelings; I just played it off. Afterwards, I immediately transferred to a different route, so that I didn't have to face him anymore and let him down.

After having been overlooked and unappreciated by my employer, I never let this affect my attitude towards them, or my strong work ethics, and the respectful and dignified way that I treated both them and my customers. One of the main reasons why was because I was living my life to please someone much greater and higher than them, which was God.

Conquering Evil with Good

Often, in order for one to be successful or victorious in life, they must overcome obstacles and badness, by conquering evil with good.

One day, during wintertime, in the early month of January, while I was out reading meters, a light rain suddenly began to fall, which was not an uncommon occurrence for our crazy, unpredictable, Minnesota weather. Subsequently, I tried working for a while, but I was just getting too wet. So I decided to head back to my car and wait for the rain to stop. To make a long story short, the weather never got any better. So at the end of the workday, I returned back to my company's office, so that I could hand in my unfinished work, which was an extremely rare thing for me to do, seeing that I normally finished any and all work that was assigned to me.

As it turned out, at the end of that particular workday, I had read a total about 35 out of the 350 or so meters in the route, which was a perfectly acceptable day's work, seeing that it was both raining and that we had an inclement weather clause (set in place by the Electrical Workers Union) that protected meter readers from working in weather that is either too cold or wet. So after returning to the office, I promptly handed in my route, and then I headed for home.

The next day, when I arrived at work to pick up my work assignment for that day, I immediately noticed that something very unusual and strange was going on. Apparently, the problem was, I was assigned two routes to read, instead of just one. This was very shocking and confusing to me, seeing that no one is ever given two routes to read in one day. That's simply too much work for one person do! So I asked my supervisor if this was a mistake. To my surprise, he said: "No."

"You've got to be kidding me! How am I supposed to finish two routes?" I replied to my Supervisor.

"I don't expect you to finish them. Just go out there and do what you can," my Supervisor said, with a half grin on his face.

Knowing the personality and disposition of my boss, I quickly realized that he was deliberately being mean and unfair. So I turned and I looked at the Union Steward (who was also a meter reader too), and my fellow coworkers who happened to be in the room with me for backing and support.

Unfortunately, although the Union Steward and my fellow coworkers should have stood up for me and explained to our Supervisor that his work demands and actions with respects to me, are completely out of line; not one of them said a single word in my behalf. They just stood there, leaving me all alone to defend for myself, which left me feeling both hurt and depressed. As a matter of fact, I was so upset, that all I wanted to do is just leave and go home.

Fortunately, for me, there happened to be a secretary named Stella, at our office building, whom I felt that I could confide in and talk to, an elderly woman that I considered to be wise and insightful. So I went to her, and I told her what had happened.

When Stella heard my story, she said to me, concerning my Boss: "He's just being a jerk!"

I informed Stella that I was feeling extremely down and depressed about the situation, and that as a direct result, my morale was very low. And because of this, it most likely will affect my work production that day. I told her that when I get out to the route, I'm thinking about just dragging my feet and not reading very many meters. However, Stella quickly cautioned me not to do this. She said I would just be playing into my Supervisor's hands.

"That's exactly what he wants you to do, so that he can disciple you afterwards for it!" Stella said.

Stella then recommended a solution to handling the problem. She said that I should go out onto the route and do the exact opposite, and work as hard as I can. She said: "If you do this, it will help you to forget about what happened. And you will have a better day!"

I thought about it for a moment. And then I said to Stella: "That's very good advice, Stella! I'm going to do exactly what you said! Thank you so much for your help!" Afterwards, I promptly left the office, and I went out into the work field to read meters.

To make a long story short, when I got out into the work field, I ran so hard and so fast, that I finished not one, but both routes! And not only that, I finished both of them within the timeframe of about six hours. That's the completion of two routes in less than one work day!

The secretary was right! I not only felt better, but I also forgot about the problem. And I had a great day!

At the end of the day, I was very proud of myself for having achieved such an amazing feat! But not only that, because of having field release, which meant that I was able to go straight home afterwards; I did not have to report back to my company until the next day. The funny thing is, as I was driving home from work that day, I could just imagine my Supervisor waiting at the office until 5:00 pm or later, for me to return with a lot of unfinished work. However, the joke was on him! Because I didn't have to return after all — a thought that personally brought me an elated sense of joy and satisfaction, knowing that he expected me to have a miserable day.[37]

The next day when I arrived at work, I proudly walked into the meter reading office, and straight up to my Supervisor who was seated at his desk, and I placed both of the routes that he had assigned me to work the previous day, down in front of him, and then I turned and immediately walked out of the room.

As soon as I left the room, one of my fellow coworkers came running up behind me. And he said to me with a very anxious and worried tone of voice: "What did you do? Did you finish both of those routes?"

"Yep," I replied.

"Why did you do that? Do you know what this is going to do to the rest us?" he said, with a highly disturbed and upset voice.

In response, I said to him: "Where were you and the others

---

[37] A regular workday for meter readers was 8 hours long; from 8:00 am to 5:00 pm (not including an hour for lunch). However, because we had field release, if we happened to finish our route early, than we could go directly home afterwards, and not have to report back to the office until the next workday. However, if we didn't finish the entire route we could not go directly home, but instead we were required to bring the unfinished portion of the work back to the office by the end of the workday, which was 5:00 pm.

yesterday, when I needed your help then? Not even one of you backed me up, or spoke up for me when I needed you most. You didn't speak up and tell our boss that it was wrong and unfair for him to give me *two routes* to work in one day!"

After listening to what I said, there was nothing that my fellow coworker could say, because he knew that I was right. Afterwards, I turned and left, and I walked into the employee lunch and break room, and over to a vending machine to get a cup of hot chocolate.

As I stood at the vending machine, my Supervisor entered the room, and he walked up to me, and said: "Chuck, can I speak to you for a moment?"

"Sure," I replied. Afterwards, both he and I sat down at a table nearby.

"Chuck, I wanted to tell you that you did a fantastic job yesterday! I didn't expect you to finish *both* routes!" my Supervisor said with both a shocked and impressed look on his face.

"I know you didn't," I replied, with a solemn tone in my voice, and a serious look on my face. And then, I promptly got up from the table; went in and retrieved my route for that workday, and left.

Later, when I told Stella (the secretary who had earlier given me the great advice) what had happened, we both had the biggest laugh! However, unfortunately, sometime later, because my boss continued to single me out and cause problems for me, I had to both report and take him before the Electrical Workers Union for further discriminatory actions against me, which he eventually got reprimanded for.

Mom Passes Away

Sadly, in the autumn of 1997, my beloved mother died from breast cancer. She was seventy three years old at the time. Her passing was a devastating blow to me, not only because she meant so much to me, but also because she was the only sure thing that made true sense in my life. She was my "Rock of Gibraltar," my "Bright Shining Star," the one that held things together for me in a cold, cruel, troubled, and racially divided world.

Initially, when mom died, for some reason I couldn't cry. However, the stress associated with it built up and grew so much, that eventually I felt like my head was going to explode from the sheer pressure. Subsequently, one day, while I was going for an early morning walk (about 5:00 am), and reflecting on what had happened, my legs collapsed, and I fell to the ground upon my knees. And I finally broke down and cried.

Later, at Mom's funeral, which was attended by a huge crowd of family and friends, I was privileged to give the eulogy. And, although I was a trained and polished public speaker, it was the hardest thing that I had ever been called on to do in my entire life. However, I must have done a pretty good job, because a lot of people said that they liked it. Even the funeral home director himself approached and told me that it was the best eulogy that he had ever heard!

A Non-Supportive Workplace

Unfortunately, when mom died, my job at the Electric Company (where, at the time, I had worked for 18 years), didn't even have the decency of giving or mailing me a sympathy card. As a matter of fact (although they were totally aware of her death) they didn't even acknowledge that she had died. How sad!

To add insult to injury, shortly after mom died, a father of one of my fellow meter readers (a Caucasian man), also died. When my job learned of it, they immediately took up a collection of money for him. Afterwards, they gave it to him, along with a sympathy card, and they told him that they were very sorry for his lost! Now, although this was a nice and supportive thing that my company did for my fellow coworker, I thought it was very discriminatory, and a cruel thing that they didn't do the same thing for me. The truth is, I would have been happy to receive just an acknowledgement and sympathy card, because at least this would have shown that they somewhat cared.

Unfortunately, this was not the first and only time that something like this happened to me in life. It also happened about 29 years earlier, when I was in the sixth grade. The incident was this: As it so happened, the father of a boy (a Caucasian kid) in my class died. So my teacher and the class took up a collection for him, and gave it to him, along with a sympathy card. They also let him stand up in front of the class and relate to us how much his father had meant to him, which I thought was a pretty nice thing for the teacher and class to do.[38]

Sad to say however, a short time later, within the same school year and class, my father died from leukemia. But for me, the teacher and class took up no collection. And neither did they give me a sympathy card. And then, to add insult to injury, one day, my teacher (a Caucasian woman) pulled me aside, and she said to me: "Charles, we [her and my fellow students] didn't take up a collection for you when your father died, because you don't live with your father."

Wow, what a cold and gut wrenching thing for a young person to have to experience! Although, I was only about 12 years old at the time, I remember that this insensitive an unjust treatment was extremely hurtful to me. Because, even though my father and mother were separated and divorced, he was still my father. And I loved and missed him just as much, if not even more than the white kid loved and missed his father.

Many years later, as I look back now, I think that this and the many other unjust and hurtful race related experiences that I went

---

[38] The school year was 1967-68, when segregation was being incorporated and enforced in schools for the first time in the United States. And when American Civil Rights Activist and Leader, Martin Luther King Jr. was brutally assassinated on April 4, 1968.

through in life played an important factor and big part in my depression and eventual mental breakdown. Because, instead of being forgiving, forgetting, and putting these things behind me, I chalked them up as cruel acts of injustice and racism — problems that I let stew and build up, and eat away at me, until eventually, they, along with many other additional and accumulative future problems became too much of a load or heavy burden for me to bear. And then, finally, one day, the last problem became the straw that broke the camel's back so to speak. True, the human mind is an amazing, adaptable, and resilient thing. But sometimes it can only take so much emotional pain and abuse!

Now that I am older and wiser, I have come to learn that it is much better to forgive, rather than keep account of the injuries that people might inflict on us. In addition to this the Bible encourages us to leave things in God's hands. For he tells us at Romans chapter 12 and verse 9: "Do not avenge yourselves, beloved, but yield place to the wrath; for it is written: "'Vengeance is mine; I will repay.'" If only I had known and applied this earlier in my life. It could have possibly saved me a lot of heartache and pain.

Another important thing to consider is that as limited creatures, we often don't have control over many of the things that happen to us in life. But we do have control over how we personally view matters and how we let them affect us. Interestingly, in the Bible, the man who lived in ancient times named Job, who suffered many tragedies, and as a result, whose wife said to him: "Curse God and die!" Replied to her: "You are talking like one of the senseless women. Should we accept only what is good from the true God and not accept also what is bad?" (Job 2:9) Like Job, I now truly believe that this is the healthier and best outlook to have on life and the things that we experience, because it can serve as a protection for both us and our families in many ways.

Further Coping with the "False Image"

Although meter readers daily and regularly worked alone, without having to spend much time with fellow coworkers, there were occasions when we were forced to spend time together. For the most part this happened only when there was inclement weather conditions, such as rain, freezing cold, etc., which according to a weather clause that was negotiated and put in place by our Local Electrical Workers Union; prohibited us from working. Basically, the clause stipulated that meter readers did not have to work under certain bad weather conditions such as in the rain, or if the temperature was colder than -10 degrees below Fahrenheit (-12.22 degrees Celsius) in the winter. During these unfavorable conditions we had to just sit at the office during the workday, either until the weather improved, or at the end of the workday.

One day, because the weather was inclement, several meter readers and I were sitting at a large table in the conference room of our meter reading office, chatting with one another. At the time, one of the guys (a Caucasian man) was relating to the group his personal interests and life pursuits. The truth is, he was a pretty smart guy who had a lot of knowledge. And because of this he was noted for always talking about some intellectual things of personal interest.

When the man was finished speaking, another meter reader, who was also Caucasian, and who was sitting directly across from me, turned, and he looked directly at me. Then, he smiled, and in a belittling and taunting tone, he said to me: "I bet you wish that you could do that?" In other words, he was implying that I lacked both the capability and intelligence to comprehend and accomplish anything that his fellow white friend could do.

In reply, I said to him: "I too have an interest in many educational fields of study, and so forth." But of course, he didn't believe me. He just sat there with a smirk on his face, rolling his eyes in disbelief, as if to say: *"Oh yeah, sure!"*

Normally, in the past, I wouldn't have said anything in reply to the man, or to anyone else for that matter. But because my mom had recently died from breast cancer, which was a pretty heavy blow to me; I had finally grown tire of just quietly sitting back and putting up with people and their negative stereotyping, demoralizing insults, and unjust mistreatment, etc. And from that time forward I had resolved and vowed within myself to stand up for myself and fight back.

So I calmly stood up and I walked over to the man that made the belittling, smart remark to me. And I proceeded to point my finger at the back of his head, at the location of his brainstem. Then I said to him: "Some people have a dysfunctional reticular formation!"[39] In response, the man looked up at me from his chair with a wide-eyed, shocked, and puzzled look on his face. And he said to me: "What does that mean? Wait a minute... are you saying that I'm brain-dead?"

"Some people are!" I replied. And then I turned and walked away.

From that day forward, neither he, nor anyone else for that matter, dared to question my intelligence, nor did they ever ridicule me again.

Emergence of a New Identity

After my mother died, I started writing poems, which is something that I had never done before. As a matter of fact, I didn't even know that I had the gift or ability to do this. And what's even stranger is that prior to this, I didn't even have the desire or intention to ever write. But not only that, I was 41 years old at the time.

Because thoughts and poems came to me randomly and during

---

[39] The reticular formation is located in the human brainstem. It consists of a tiny network of nerves that is the size of a person's little finger. It acts like a traffic control center that monitors the flow of millions of messages that flow into the brain through the senses. Its function or job is to quickly sort through the avalanche of incoming information, sorting out the trivial and selecting the essential. Each second it permits only a few hundred at most to enter the cerebral cortex or conscience mind.

unexpected times, I had to start carrying around an ink pen and pocket notepad, so that I could quickly jot them down, otherwise they could have been so easily forgotten and lost forever, which was a painful thing that I experienced many times in the past.

I even kept a notebook and pen next to my bed at night. But this soon became an annoyance to my wife, who was trying to sleep, because I would frequently turn the nightstand light on and off again, so that I could see to record my thoughts. Finally, she said to me: "I'm trying to sleep. But I can't if you're going to keep doing that! You're going to have to sleep on the couch!" So I would get up, go into the other room, lie down, and repeat the same process. At least this time I was not disturbing my wife's valuable sleep.

When it comes to traveling on the road of life, sometimes it can take an unexpected turn, or it takes us on a route or path in a completely different direction and in ways that we would never have expected. Personally, I found this to be true in my case. Because after my mother died, I became or transformed into a completely different person. I think the main reason why is because during that particular somber and sad time in my life, I had become very dissatisfied with the person that I had become. It's not that I was a bad person or anything, or that I was a complete and utter failure. For overall, I was a pretty good and respected person—one who had gained a certain measure of success in life. The problem was, I was angry that I had allowed society and the world around me to greatly shape and influence the person that I had ultimately become. In other words, I felt that life had robbed me of my true nature, character, and identity, and of some of the more important things about myself that were being left undiscovered.

Interestingly, the depression that I was undergoing, which was being induced or brought on by my beloved mother's death, along with periods of isolation and self reflection, allowed me to delve deep within myself — to discover and uncover the true, hidden person that lies within — a person that possessed certain abilities and talents that I never knew existed before, prior to this time. And these were beginning to slowly emerge and come forward.

In the past, prior to my mom's passing, I was primary an athlete and physical person. Some of the things that I regularly pursued were: I loved to exercise, to jog, to do weight training at the health club 4 to 5 days a week, to play basketball, tennis, touch football, softball, to watch sporting events on TV, as well as attending them in person, etc. Yep, when it came to exercise and sports, I just couldn't seem to get enough!

But after taking a good and hard look at the person that I was inside, I quickly left all of these things behind. And I started to do other things instead — things that I believed were more in tune with my true character, soul, and being... and that I personally felt were more self-rewarding and valuable.

Another curious and interesting thing, is that I personally feel and believe that sometimes, because some people are so distinct and different from others, and they don't seem to fit into a certain structure or mold within society or elsewhere, or they happen to be lost in the world and can't find themselves (their true character and identity), that this causes them to feel sad, which can lead to more serious forms of depression, and even bipolar disorder if left unchecked.

Metamorphic Transformation

Shedding my old personality, along with discovering the different and exciting new individual in me, was a slow, gradual, and progressive process and experience. As a matter of fact, I am still learning new things about myself every day!

Some of the things that I was now pursing and doing, which I had never done before in the past, were: writing poetry, short stories and novels; learning to play a musical instrument; and composing original music and writing songs.

The interesting thing is, when I began doing many of these

things, I was forty one years old at the time.

In addition to discovering that I have a natural knack for writing poetry, I purchased a Roland XP80 electronic keyboard/music station, which initially I didn't know how to play. And I began learning and teaching myself how to play, compose, and record my own original music. Wow, what a big difference this was from the person that I was in the past! Because prior to this time, I had never written or composed any songs before.

The reason why I got interested in music composition is because throughout my life I have always heard and created music in my head. And now, finally, I wanted to see if I could reproduce the sounds and songs that I was hearing, and play them on an actual keyboard. The crazy thing is, I thought that this was the way it was for all people in general — that everyone had the ability to hear and create music in their heads. However, I soon found out from a real or actual musician, that not everyone is able to do this. And that what I was experiencing was due to having a special and innate, God-given gift. I don't know if this is true, but, all I can say is that I was now having the time of my life!

Initially, when I first began music composition, it was something that was really hard to do. But as time progressed it got a little easier day by day. Today, I still struggle with it somewhat, but the rewards of listening to the end results of making and producing songs can be a lot of fun. Sure, I may not be a Mozart, Beethoven, Bach, Bob James, Stevie Wonder, or Prince, but at least I have the enjoyment and satisfaction that comes from being able to express my own individual creativity.

Another thing that I've discovered is that I have a love for writing. So far I have written five books, all of which have been published, including this one that you are reading now.

To tell you the truth, I honestly believe that all humans have the ability to do these things, and much, much, more! It all depends on what we happen to be exposed to and what appeals to us personally. Sure, it may be a little more challenging for some of us, especially if we are starting or trying new things for the first time, or if we get started later in life, or if we happen to have certain handicaps or problems. But it definitely can be done, as is shown in my case, and many others.

When I think about the new, real, and exciting individual that I recently have been discovering in me, I can't help but to think about the "false image" of the 'Negro' that was created through slavery, and how it has destroyed so many black people's lives throughout American history, down to the present day. And it makes me feel sad. However, today, because we as individuals exercise a certain degree of power and influence over our own lives, it's important for us to take advantage of this, so that we become masters of our own fate so to speak, rather than forfeiting or losing out on what might have been, or what we can potentially become.

Chapter 5

A NEW CAREER CHANGE

I n the year 2001, I decided to leave the electric company that I had worked at for so many years, and pursue a different employment career. This was both a big and scary move for me, because I had been a meter reader for twenty two long years. Also, I was no longer a spring chicken, for I was forty five years old at the time. Nonetheless, I felt that the most important thing was that I needed to try something new and different for a change.

At the time, I didn't know exactly what kind of new career I wanted to pursue. But because there was a high demand for jobs in the computer industry in the year 2000, I felt that perhaps I would go to college for computer science, and then get a job in that field (although I knew absolutely nothing about computers, except for turning them on, and sometimes even that simple task posed a challenge:)

To help me in my pursuit of a new career, the Electric Company, who was now my former employer, provided me with a career counselor. This is something that they were required to do by law, because of the way that I left, which is too long of a story at this time to explain.

One of the first things that my career counselor helped me with was writing a resume, which was something that I never had to use or do before. He also scheduled an appointment for me to have both an aptitude and Intelligence Quotient (IQ) test taken.

I remember the day of testing. It took all day (from 8:00 am till 5:00 pm), with only one fifteen minute break in between. Then, later, after the conclusion of the day, the tests administrator informed me that my test results would take about two weeks to process or complete. And that she will telephone me when they come in; at which time she will then schedule a date and time for me to come back into her office to discuss them.

As I drove home from the testing facility that day, I thought to myself: *"Wow, I'm going to hate to see those test results! I bet that when I return, they'll be holding up a big sign that says: 'Moron!'"*

Later, after about two weeks went by, I received a phone call. It was the test administrator. She told me that my test results are in. And then she arranged a day and time for me to meet with her at her office.

Interestingly, on the day that I walked back into the test administrator's office, to my surprise, my career counselor was also there, along with the tests administrator. But the thing that was really strange was that both of them were sitting there with big chessy cat grins on their faces, which made me feel a little awkward, curious, and wonder what the heck was going on!

After I was seated, the tests administrator informed me about my test scores. She said: "Charles, you tested really high! As a matter of fact, in the entire thirteen years that I have been testing people, no one has ever been in the upper category that you're in, nor had they scored as high as you did. You are highly intelligent!

Your intelligence level is found in only one percent of the population. And your spatial intelligence is way off the charts! You are the kind of person that makes a difference in the world!"

I thought to myself: *"Wow... what a surprise!"*

The crazy thing is, at the time of the testing, I only had a high school diploma. I didn't have a college education or vocational training or anything.

Afterwards, the tests administrator, and my career counselor, who was also amazed by my test results, told me that I have the intelligence and capabilities to pursue any job or career that I want. They said that I could be a judge, a lawyer, a doctor, a librarian, or anything that I choose to be. And then, out of curiosity, they asked me how in the world I could have read meters for 22 years, and not have gotten bored?

I assured them that I was never bored reading meters, because I was always busy. I told them that I have both a passion for and an insatiable appetite for knowledge and learning. And that because my job had field release, and I regularly finished my routes early, I would spend much of my spare time on things such as: studying and reading books on various subjects; visiting libraries; arts and science museums; discovering and enjoying a variety of music; and many other things; along with engaging in fun things with my wife and kids, such as visiting parks and lakes, and going on bike rides, etc.

I informed the tests administrator and career counselor that because I have a love for learning and books, that I would regularly check a variety of them out of the local libraries — books on various subjects such as: science, biology, human anatomy, horticulture, astronomy, history, poetry, bibliographies of famous people, Shakespearean literature, the structure and functions of the human brain, and single-celled organisms, and so forth.

I also explained to them that while I was working reading meters, that I would often carry a pocket notepad and pen with me, so that I could compose and write poetry along the way. Also, at other times, I would listen to some easy-listening, classical music by Mozart, Beethoven, Chopin, Bach, Rachmaninoff, and various other composers, on a Walkman, Compact Disk (CD) player.[40] The truth is, I was an extremely studious, highly curious, and exploitative person that had a lot of things and pursuits to keep me busy.

Interestingly (although I didn't realize it at that time); future jobs would come to love me, because I could work at and perform my job duties at very high performance levels. As a result, they could get away with underpaying me (without having to pay me top dollar), due to the reason, as they would say: "You lack required work experience," Or "You don't have certain academic credentials or degrees."

After explaining to my career counselor and the tests administrator that I was not bored reading meters, they asked me what employment career I was thinking about pursuing. I told them: "It's going to be a difficult choice, because I don't have the luxury of spending many years in college. For I have a wife and kids to financially support. Unfortunately, the most time that I can spend in school is about two years. True, I'll be receiving severance pay for a year; after having been voluntarily laid-off from work at my meter reading job. And I have a little money set aside. But this is only going to last for so long. Because of this, I will need to choose a job career that requires only a two year degree."

In addition, I also informed the tests administrator and career counselor that I needed to find a job that offered some variety, one that I would not get bored with so easily. Because there are so many jobs in the field of employment that are so repetitious and monotonous—jobs that require you to perform the same tasks over

---

[40] One of the reasons why I chose classical music to listen to is because I needed a little extra stimulus for my mind or brain while I worked. Another reason was because it wasn't as distracting as some genres of music can be. This way I could still concentrate on doing my job.

and over again, which is something that would drive me nuts! They said: "You're going to have that problem with just about any job." In reply, I said: "I realize that. But in regards to repetition, some jobs are worse than others."

Another thing I mentioned to them, was that I needed to pursue a career in a field were the demand for jobs is high, and also one that pays well. And for that reason I said: "I'm thinking about going into the field of electronics." In response, they said: "That's a good choice!"

Back to School

In January of 2002, I entered a local college for electronics. This was quite an undertaking, seeing that I hadn't been in school for such a long time. In truth, it had been over 28 years since I graduated from high school!

I remember my first day of college at the electronics institute. I was so excited! Because of my love for learning and books, I just couldn't wait to start! I was like a giddy, little kindergartener, who was going to school for the very first time, with his lunchbox in hand. Little did I realize that I would soon be in for a rude shock and awakening! Because, as it turned out, college was nothing like I had expected it to be. But rather, I found its academic structure to be downright monotonous and boring, and also the teachers to be partial and arrogant. What a big letdown! Now, instead of being like an excited kid entering a candy store or toy shop, I was returning home at the end of the day, walking slumped over with my head hanging low, and with a look of dejection on my face; dragging my lunchbox behind.

When I initially enrolled in college, I started out in the electronics day program (9:00 am to 4:00 pm). But I soon fell behind in one of the classes. It wasn't that the curriculum or information was too difficult to comprehend. But rather, it was because there were just too many daily worksheet handouts that needed to be completed and turned in ASAP. In other words, the pace was too fast, which was something that I was not use to, nor was it in alignment with my personality and my individual structure of learning and doing things.

In truth, I found this learning structure to be contrary to my way of thinking and learning. Personally, I prefer to work at my own pace, so that I can thoroughly grasp and absorb everything. I'm not satisfied with just completing and handing in senseless worksheet assignments, whether I understand them or not, which was all that the school required. Also, the school's teaching style (the way that the teachers or instructors verbally disseminated the information) was a very slow and methodical, step-by-step process, that didn't explain the big picture of *what* it was about, *why* these things were being taught, and *where* it all was headed or leading to. What a disappointment! And the surprising thing is, this school was listed and highly noted for being one of, if not the best technical schools for electronics in the entire State of Minnesota.

In addition to its overall academic structure, I also found the school's leaning environment to be too noisy, busy, and distracting—making it very hard to focus and concentrate. Subsequently, during tests, I literally had to wear earplugs, and sit at the back of the room, so that I could focus on the material at hand. Interestingly, although I didn't recognize it at the time, I now realize that this was possibly early signs of bipolar disorder, although not yet in the full-blown stage.

Because the structure of the electronics day school program was not to my liking, after finishing the first semester, I dropped out of the program, and I began attending the night school program instead. And although this offered only an electronics diploma, instead of a degree, I felt that overall it was a much better fit. Besides, at that time, I also came to learn that an electronics diploma is all that one needs to get a decent paying job in the electronics field. And that an electronics diploma in comparison to a degree, is about the same, as far as gaining decent employment in the field of electronics is concerned. Also, in the diploma program, academically, you're learning the exact, same things that are being taught in the degree program, but at a much cheaper price. Overall, the diploma program was about $10,000.00 dollars cheaper than the degree program. That's a lot of money saved!

Additional benefits of attending night school was that it afforded me the opportunity of working part-time during the day as an electronic technician for a low-voltage lighting company, where I gained valuable work experience, along with earning some additional money to help support my family while I was in school.

Dealing with Prejudice in College

Unfortunately, overall, when it came to teaching, I found that most of my college instructors lacked true teaching abilities. They personally thought that they were great, but this was just the effects of having overly inflated egos. However, I did find one of the teachers in particular to have a very special gift. As it so happens, he was a retired medical engineer; a self-made millionaire, named Mr. Gamble.[41]

It wasn't Mr. Gamble prominence or money that made him unique and special, but rather it was his knack for making the difficult easy to comprehend. And also for making the learning experience an enjoyable one.

Oddly and unconventionally, during the first two weeks of class, Mr. Gamble didn't teach us electronics at all. But instead, he just focused solely on physics, which I found to be absolutely fascinating! Interestingly, much of what he was teaching, I had already learned about in my personal reading and studies that I did in the past, during the time I was a meter reader. As he lectured to the class, I would frequently intervene, which he didn't seem to mind at all. And I would carry on short conversations with him about the subjects at hand.

One day, during breaktime, Mr. Gamble told me that I didn't belong in the electronics program. He said that I was too smart for

---

[41] The name has been changed.

this. He said that I needed to be in an engineering college instead; one that contained heavy subject matter, where I would be more intellectually challenged. I thanked him for the complement, but then, I informed him that I didn't have the luxury of spending four years or more in college, because I have a wife and kids to support and provide for, and for that reason, I chose a two year electronics course, instead of four years.

Unfortunately, the other teachers at the electronics college were nothing like Mr. Gamble. A few of them, due to discriminatory thinking and practices, even gypped me out of A's —by the smallest and narrowest of percentage margins. One of them was so racially biased that he didn't even bother to hide his prejudice. Consequently, one day, because of the discriminate way I was being treated by him, I got up and deliberately walked out of his class—a move that shocked many of my fellow students. Interestingly, as I was leaving class, one of my classmates turned and he looked at me, and said: "Wow, you must be really smart, if you don't need the teacher?" In reply, I said to him: "Whatever he [the teacher] teaches, I can learn in the school books." And then, I promptly exited the room and went home for the day.

As it turned out, I really didn't like being in college. And if it wasn't for me being able to help fellow students by tutoring them, which was requested of me, I probably wouldn't have stayed.

Knowledge and Pain

In regards to some situations if life, what we personally don't know can't hurt us. And, sometimes the more that we know, can make matters worse. And although I believe that having a certain measure of knowledge is important, I now feel that knowledge and intelligence can sometimes be a curse, which is a pretty strange statement coming from me, considering that I have an insatiable appetite for knowledge. The reason why I feel this way is that experience has taught me that the more that you know the greater the pain that comes with it. One reason why is because we often lack the ability and power to put the wisdom or knowledge we possess to good use. Another is because it is not always appreciated and accepted by others.

An addition thing is that knowledge can make one an ugly target for persecution. For most people don't like it when you're too smart! They also don't like it when you cause waves. In my opinion, because of the suffering and pain that often comes with having knowledge, sometimes it's better to be an average Joe. This way you can be content and go through life pretty much accepting things for the way that they are, without the consequences of being frustrated and hurt by the pain and injustices that you experience or observe in the world around you.

Unfortunately, because of the "false image," which portrays blacks as being inferior to the white race, in regards to intelligence, I've often felt like I've had to prove my intelligence, especially later in life. Not necessarily to others, but to myself. Interestingly, it's been said that an intelligent person, such as a doctor, lawyer, scientist, etc., have a vocabulary of about 4000 to 5000 words. Inspired by this and wondering how large my personal vocabulary is, one day, I purchased a thick notebook, and I began to randomly write down in it all the words that came to my mind. At that particular time in my life, I had the luxury of doing this, because I was newly laid off from work and was receiving severance pay for a full year. So I took some time off before I started college in January of 2002, to take a short vacation and pursue some other things.

After jotting down many words, which took awhile, I reached 1000 words, then 2000, then 3000, and finally 5000 words. But then, suddenly, I came to my senses. As it dawned on me, I thought to myself: *"What in the world am I doing? What am I trying to prove? I don't have to prove anything to anyone! Sure, this exercise is somewhat good for my self esteem, but in reality it really doesn't matter. The important thing is that I know and that I have confidence, and that I believe in myself; that I am just as capable and intelligence as anyone else. And that I can accomplish anything that I put my heart and mind to — that's all that matters!"*

Interestingly, although I could have gone much further than I did. From then on, I laid down my notebook and pen, and completely let it go.

Sad to say, as a result of growing up in a racist society, and being viewed and treated as being intellectually inferior to the white race my entire life, I guess I felt that I had to prove to them, and also to myself to a certain degree that I wasn't (even though this wasn't necessarily done consciously at the time).

Life in the Field of Electronics

In the year 2003, I graduated from Electronics College. Now, it was time for me to find a job in my field of study. Although, during and after college I worked as an electronic technician for a couple of different companies, sometime later I was hired at a larger, more prestigious and preferred company. As a matter of fact, it is one of the largest cardiac pacemaker and defibrillator companies in the world. Believe it or not, the department that I worked in had a total of about 115 engineers and technicians!

The position that I occupied in the company, was that of being an electronic test technician in the Test Engineering Department. The thing that I liked most about the job was that I was not micromanaged. But rather, I was treated as a responsible adult and worker. All I was required to do was to report to my project manager once a week; update him on how things were going on the job, and that was it.

Another interesting thing about my job was that my work environment was unique and unusual, in that, even though I was only an electronic technician, I was working in the engineering department alongside of electronic engineers, and also actual medical doctors (something that other technicians were not allowed to do). As a matter of fact, I personally had a large work cubicle that was situated right within the heart and midst of them. The reason I was there, is because I was hired as a contract worker to work on a special project. The job was to last only six months, with the possibility of being hired permanently at the end of that time period.

As it turned out, my project manager, who was also an engineer by profession; was given an extremely important and pressing job assignment by the big director of the test engineering group. It was a Remedial Action (RMA) project that was being demanded and driven by the Food and Drug Administration (FDA). Apparently, the purpose of the project was to fix or clean up some internal problems that where associated with the company's test documents, so as to be in total compliance with FDA regulations.

As it so happened, I and two other electronic technicians were temporarily hired to work on the RMA project together, which required that we first get certified. This involved a lot of training and tests that we were required to pass. But it also required that we become familiar with the company's electronic test equipment, machines, and written procedures, which were used for building cardiac pacemakers and defibrillators. In all, we were given two months to get certified and up to date on everything.

Wasting no time at all, I poured myself into the huge task. The reason being is that I wanted to get certified and approved ASAP. Interestingly, to my project manager's surprise, I completed everything within one week! Now, I was thoroughly ready, eager, and certified to take on the big RMA project.

To my dismay, however, when it came time to actually begin the RMA project, neither I nor my fellow coworkers were given any instructions from management on how to start, carry out or proceed with the actual project. The reason why is because there wasn't any! As it so happened, my project manager didn't really know what he was doing. He had absolutely no clue on how to perform an RMA. Apparently, this was the first time that an RMA project was done at the company, and so there was no written procedure for it.

As time went by, I was becoming increasingly impatient and

tired of just sitting there waiting for instructions and direction to come from my boss or upper management. So I decided to go ahead of him and get the project rolling.

What I did was I personally took it upon myself to figure out everything that was needed and required to thoroughly perform and complete an RMA project. Then I wrote and provided the company with the step-by-step, written instructions and procedures (which ended up being a thirteen page document), for carrying out the entire RMA process from start to finish. Afterwards, I emailed it to my project manager. And I asked him if I could share this information with my fellow coworkers (the other two contract employees that were hired along with me to work on the RMA project).[42]

The very moment that my project manager received my documented RMA instructions and procedures, he was absolutely ecstatic and thrilled! Because, now, my fellow coworkers and I could proceed with the project, and perhaps get it done within the allotted six month deadline that we were given by the FDA. To make a long story short, in the end, as it turned out, we not only completed the project, but we also got it done two to three weeks early!

What is interesting is that when I wrote the RMA instructions and procedures, I arranged or set up the entire document in easy to read and follow table format. To my surprise, as it turned out, this type of document formatting style is something that was not seen or used by the company before, in regards to how they format their own internal documents and written manufacturing instructions and procedures. And when one of the technical writers for the test engineering group, who had a degree in journalism seen what I had done, he said to me: "We [the company] never use table format in our documents!" However, shortly thereafter, the company quickly adopted this table format style and began to set up and format their

---

[42] After I emailed my manager my written RMA instructions and procedures, he told me to immediately email copies of this to my fellow coworkers, which I did. And, like my boss, they too were appreciative and happy to receive them.

documents this same way.

In the end, for getting the big RMA project done, my project manager was given rave reviews and a lot of praise by the big Test Engineering Group Director (who assigned him the job), and many other coworkers.

Extremely grateful for what I had done; my project manager thanked me several times privately for voluntarily taking an important lead in the RMA project, and for writing and providing the needed instructions and procedures, etc. Sure, in the end he got all of the credit for completing this important and pressing FDA driven project. But, I ended up with a steady, fulltime job. For the company hired me on as a permanent employee right after this. As it turned out, I was hired to work as an electronic test technician on the third or graveyard shift. Of course, I would have preferred a job on first or day shift, but apparently there wasn't anything available for me at the time.

Taking Credit for Another Man's Work

Unfortunately, I soon found out that working third shift was pretty tuff, especially because my wife was beginning to undergo some serious health problems. And because of this she preferred me to be home at night. Luckily for both of us, after about a year, I was able to transfer to a different job within the company that was on first shift — working as an Electronic Quality Technician on the Material Review Board (MRB) in the pacemaker and defibrillator manufacturing department.[43] My job was to find product electrical failures, and catch and stop them before product was completely built, released, sold, and implanted in cardiac patients.

On a daily basis I would work both hard and fast. On average, I

---

[43] The Material Review Board is a committee of people who collect and discuss the outcome and treatment of product or material that has been labeled nonconforming (in regards to product requirements), so as to prevent unintended use or delivery.

would get all of my work done within about four or five hours or so. Afterwards, I would ask my manager if he had more work for me to do.

One day, when my manager found out that I have both a love for and also the ability to write, he had me get certified to process Change Orders (CO)—something that I happily agreed to do. CO's for the most part were in-house, regulatory projects that engineers primarily worked on. The purpose of COs was for making changes or improvements in such things as: test equipment, products, and written manufacturing documents and procedures, etc.

After getting CO certified, which involved a considerable amount of learning, study, and testing (in addition to doing my regular daily work assignments in MRB); one highly important project that I was given to do, involved an urgent issue that was FDA demanded and driven. Unfortunately, it involved a serious problem that occurred in the past, in regards to our company's oversight and negligence.

Sad to say, the problem was that eight cardiac patients or customers who had our company's Implantable Cardioverter Defibrillators (ICD) implanted in them, died, due to product failures.[44] Apparently, these tragedies took place about three or four years prior to me receiving the important work assignment. As a result, FDA shut us down, and our company was not allowed to build and sale anymore of that particular defibrillator product line until the problem was completely resolved and fixed. In addition to this, in the event that when and if the problem did get fixed, our company was then also required at that time to prove to both the FDA and the Medicines and Healthcare products Regulatory Agency (MHRA), that our product is now perfectly safe, and that it no longer poses any dangerous health risks. Yes, it was an extremely huge deal, to say the least![45]

---

[44] An Implantable Cardioverter Defibrillator is a medical device that is surgically implanted in the chest or abdomen of a patient. It works to reset an abnormal heartbeat back to normal.

[45] The Medicines and Healthcare products Regulatory Agency is an executive

Since human error played a substantial role or factor in the defibrillator failures, my company sought to eliminate the human aspect of the building process, by automating a certain portion of the manufacturing process, which involved identifying and catching product electrical failures in advance. But this was easier said than done.[46]

Interestingly, prior to my receiving this FDA driven project (which required me to perform a lot of hard work and many complicated procedures — details of which I cannot relate, due to company privacy clauses); many others had tried hard to get it done in the years before me, which included electronic engineers, and managers. But, because of the sheer difficulty of the project and the work involved, not one of them could resolve and complete it. As a result, about 3 or 4 years had passed by; and it still was not done! As a matter of fact, the project was so difficult, troublesome, and unique, that my manager even referred to it as "The White Elephant."

At the time that I took over this huge FDA project, my project manager, who was an electronic engineer by profession, had been working on the difficult assignment himself; and he was having an extremely difficult time getting it done. While working on the project, he had even personally applied for and was granted thirteen time extensions by upper management. But now, they had finally grown impatient, and they we're not going to allow him anymore extensions.

To my surprise, shortly after I received the FDA project, I recognized that my company (others who had the project prior to me) had been going in the wrong direction with it! Once I figured this important part out, and how to proceed with the project, etc., I was able to both complete it and get it approved by the FDA and MHRA, all within the matter of a short time span of about one to two months. In response, my manager, his boss, and upper management were absolutely ecstatic and thrilled! They were so happy that this huge and difficult project was finally completed! Because, now they were out of the woods with the FDA. But also, they could finally start building their defibrillator product line once again, without harm or threat to future customers!

Upon completion of the job, my manager personally and privately thanked and praised me for completing the important FDA driven project, which apparently ended up saving his job. Confiding in me, he told me that upper management had given him a final deadline, and that they had even seriously threatened to fire him if the project wasn't completed on time. Because, even though I was personally working on the project, he as my manager was still the one that was responsible for it. What's interesting and good is that I completed the project about a month before his deadline passed.

One of the electronic engineers in my department and work group, who was highly impressed by what I had did and accomplished, in regards to the complexity and difficulty of the work assignment, and the timely completion of this extremely important FDA driven project, sad to me: "Wow Chuck, what you did was amazing! I wish I was you when it comes to work performance review time! You're going to get a big promotion and pay raise!"

Unfortunately, the sad thing is, when it came time for giving out promotions and raises, I was completely passed over. Rather than properly and rightfully rewarding me for the difficult and outstanding job that I had done, my manager and company gave my promotion and raise to one of my fellow coworkers (a Caucasian man), instead — an electronic technician who had previously worked on the project, along with an engineer, about three years prior to me. The crazy thing is, the work that the technician performed amounted to practically nothing at all. But, not only that, he and others surely did not get the difficult project done, which was proven. Nevertheless, he was rewarded with a large pay raise and promotion, something that even highly puzzled other fellow coworkers. Because they knew that he didn't do anything in particular or spectacular on the job to rightfully earn it.

To tell you the truth, this wasn't the first time that someone else in the company was given the credit for my hard work and accomplishments — which was a practice that I now realized had become a regular pattern or thing.

Throughout my life, one thing in particular that has been highly disturbing and hurtful to me, is society's refusal to acknowledge my intelligence, or achievements, especially in regards to giving me the appropriate recognition and credit when due.

Later, when I complained to upper management (my manager's boss) about the situation, and suggested to him that perhaps I should take the matter to our company's Human Resources (HR) Department. My manager's boss said: "Oh no, we don't need to go to HR! I'll take care of it."[47]

Interestingly, a couple of days later; after I got back from a short vacation that I had taken; my boss's manager approached me and informed me that my manager had immediately resigned or stepped down from being the manager of my work group. He said that my manager told him that he wanted to go back to being just an engineer, instead of being a manager, because he missed it so much! The crazy thing is, not only did they give him a job as an electronic engineer, but they also immediately moved him (before I came back to work) to a different department within the company.

---

[47] Unbeknown to upper management, prior to my speaking to my manager's boss, I had already emailed detailed information to our company's Vice President of HR about the huge FDA driven project that I was given to work on and had successfully completed. Interestingly, the way that I presented the information to him was in a sort of For Your Information (FYI) way... Telling him that I was both honored and proud to have been placed in charge of getting this most urgent and important project done.

Unfortunately, as far as the situation turned out for me, I never did receive a promotion or pay raise, nor even a simple apology.

The sad thing is, as far as work performance goes, I pretty much walked on water for my employer — by accomplishing the unthinkable! Not just this one time only, for there were other times as well. And yet, they still chose not to reward me for my high work performance and outstanding achievements.

Knowledge Is Power?

It's been said that knowledge is power. But in reality I find that this is not always true. For sometimes knowledge can leave you feeling the exact opposite, *powerless*. For example, you could be the smartest person on the planet, but if you lack the ability to put your knowledge to good use, or if you or others don't personally benefit from it, what good is it? Also, due to greed, one's knowledge can be exploited, abused, and taken advantage of by others, leaving the person totally powerless to do anything about it, as was experienced in my case. So in retrospect, as far as it goes, I've learned that the knowledge that one possesses can and will remain ineffective and powerless to a certain degree.

Knowledge can also torment one's mind and soul. In other words, sometimes a person can be too smart for their own good. For example, in the past, it was once taught and believed that the earth was the center of the universe. However, Italian astronomer, mathematician, and physicist, Galileo Galilei' (1564-1642) newly developed telescope, and his amazing scientific discoveries, clearly disproved this. As a result, he quickly made enemies amongst Catholic Theologians. In the end, the Roman Catholic Church viewed his discoveries as heresy, and as a result, he was forced to recant his findings. And he had to spend the rest of his life under house arrest.

From Galileo's example and experience we learn several things about knowledge. One thing is that knowledge can be completely useless, if others are not willing to acknowledge and accept it. And two, that sometimes having too much knowledge or intelligence can be self defeating, and even destructive. And three, that knowledge can create enemies. The truth is, sometimes we can observe, uncover, or know too much for our own good. For example, if one doesn't know that something is wrong, they most likely will have the tendency to go along with it and accept it. However, when their eyes become opened so-to-speak, in regards to seeing and recognizing the real truth of a matter; chances are they are most likely going to reject it and push for change, which many times is neither wanted nor received well by others. This is a fact no matter how well and tactful we may present or make known our valuable insight, thoughts, or ideas to others.

In the past, it used to be highly frustrating and upsetting to me when I had accurate knowledge about a subject or things that others stubbornly refused to acknowledge or accept, even though they knew that what I was saying was factual and correct. As a result, I often would double down and pushback even harder, trying to cram it down their throats so to speak. But to my chagrin, I soon discovered that this untactful approach, often, only makes matters much worse. And that if you want to promote peace and happiness you can't always live your life going against the grain. True, when it comes to things or matters of great importance that we personally may have discovered or know — that can possibly be used to advance knowledge and truth, sometimes we are left with no choice but to stick to our guns and fight for improvements or change. However, if the matter is not a life or death issue, or extremely important, sometimes it's best not to push the envelope, but instead to just let it go. It's not that you compromise who you are or what you believe in, it's just that you simply choose not to cause waves, or you prefer not to burden yourself with further frustration and pain.

When it comes to the pursuit of knowledge, I used to crave and desire it so much, that I had an insatiable appetite for it. Now, to a certain degree, I have come to loathe it. The reason why is because sometimes knowledge can cause so much frustration and pain. Interestingly, this agrees with a statement that is found in the Bible at Ecclesiastes 1:18. There, wise King Solomon of ancient times said: "An abundance of wisdom brings an abundance of frustration… [and] whoever increases knowledge increases pain."

Personally, sometimes I feel that, rather than acquiring knowledge, that perhaps it's better to be an ordinary, "Average Joe" instead. Because the more that you know, the worse things can get for you. Also, many times, what you don't know can't hurt or bother you emotionally and mentally. In this regards, you could say that "Ignorance is bliss!"

Knowledge verses Ignorance

Although, a certain amount of benightedness or lack of knowledge can be advantageous at times, on the other hand, total ignorance can be debilitating and downright dangerous. For it can put a person in harm's way, by allowing them to walk blindly into a dangerous situation or a trap. Also, if a person does not know the true value of something, they can easily be mislead, swindled or cheated.

Ignorance can also produce a sort of blinded complacency in people. In that it keeps them content with their present lot in life or place in the world, even though situations or conditions may not be the best for them or the most ideal. As a result of being stooped in ignorance, there is little chance that they will form a rebellion or push or fight for change. That is one of the reasons why slaves or black people during the time of institutional slavery in North America were denied an education. Forced ignorance was used as an effective tool to keep them blinded, content, and under total control.

So from what we just considered, we can see that knowledge is not absolute or all-powerful. However, it can be useful, good, and provide us with a relative amount of help, protection, and freedom. We also learn, in respects to ignorance, that although some may feel that there appears to be some minor benefits to being uneducated, or to be, not "in the know" (perhaps feeling that this frees them from guilt or responsibility), that total ignorance can be extremely debilitating and harmful. With this in mind, I would have to say that if it ever came down to having the choice of whether to choose *knowledge* or *ignorance*; personally, I'd choose knowledge, by far!

Release It and Let It Go

The false teaching and notion that the black race is not equal to the white race in intelligence, has never sat well with me. It has always been highly troubling and bothersome to me — like a sharp thorn in my side. But even more disturbing, is when white people don't see or acknowledge you for the true person that you are. But instead, they lower your personal value or worth, and paint you as being something completely different, which often is a person that is beneath them in all respects — inferior to them in intelligence, ability, spirituality, morality, physical cleanliness, and so forth. The sad thing is, even when you convincingly prove your equality to them, many still blatantly and stubbornly refuse to accept and acknowledge it. And what's even worse, is the more that you prove it, the more agitated and angry they often become with you. I think the reason why is because for the first time in their lives, it makes them start to feel inferior. And that doesn't make them feel good about themselves, especially when in all assumed reality, they are supposed to be (intellectually, etc) superior to you. Another reason why is because it can be hard for people to accept the truth. This reminds me of a poem that I once wrote. It is entitled, *"The Truth Hurts."* It goes like this:

The truth is hidden behind a thin veneer,

Facing exposure becomes a constant fear

Once again the veil of secrecy gets lifted away,

For agitation and insecurity ensues—the hoax betrays!

And so we rise to do battle with the sworn enemy,

To quickly relieve the hurt we perceive mentally

Unleashing multiple weapons of a diabolical state,

To vanquish exposers of the false image we create

Eagerly fighting to conceal the self inflicted shame,

Than deny the lie that brings self gratifying fame.

~

In other words, for some people, when they finally see or actually come to realize and recognize for the first time in their lives that a certain person or others don't fit a certain stereotype, other than the "false image" that they are so use to identifying with; this doesn't sit well with them. So in return, they put up a strong defense, and fight against it all the more, especially if they feel that they have something to lose.[48]

I'm not stating this to elevate them or myself above others. And I don't know why it is. But one positive and useful feature, characteristic or trait of those who are bipolar is that by nature they often are very gifted, creative, smart or intelligent people. Personally, I feel that there is nothing that I can't do, learn, or accomplish, if I focus my mind and heart on it. And, because of this, I find that this makes some white people in particular, feel very uncomfortable, and even irritable and angry with me. Interestingly, this mostly happens with those who are considered by society to be highly intelligent. As a result, academically, these one's often think that I'm stirring up rivalry or competition with them, or that I'm showing off the wisdom and knowledge I possess, or that I'm trying to make them look bad or stupid, or something. But this isn't true. I just love to learn and freely share my discoveries and knowledge with others. It makes me feel good. After all, even the Bible says: "There is more happiness in giving than there is in receiving." (Acts 20:35)

As regards 20/20 hindsight, now that I ponder and look back at

---

[48] Although this isn't the sole or only meaning or application of my poem, it serves well in helping to explain how some people react when the truth is uncovered that they are trying to ignore or hide.

the past, I'm beginning to believe that in the case of my missed job promotion at the pacemaker and defibrillator company, that a certain portion of it had to do with the jealousy and pride of others.[49] For at that time, I was only an electronic technician, with only a few years of experience under my belt. And, here I come along, and complete an extremely difficult task (in record setting time), a project that others, with more intelligence, academic accolades, knowhow, and experience, couldn't even come close to finishing. To them, they probably thought: *"How in the world can a lowly electronic technician, with only an electronics diploma, be smarter than us? But not only that, he's making us look bad!"* Subsequently, as a result, they ended up stealing what was rightfully mine.

Another possible reason or explanation for others taking the credit for my work, is that unfortunately we live in a brutal and cutthroat "dog-eat-dog world," where many people will do just about anything and everything that they can to advance to the top, or to gain something that they deem valuable in the process, including stealing or taking credit for another man's work.

Today, although I truly have just cause or reason to be angry with my job and certain people for how they treated me in the past — now, since that time, I find that the best thing for me to do, is just to forgive, release it, and let it go. For it will do me no good to just sit around and stew about it. This would only cause me further harm and pain.

Educational Requirements Today

Unlike the insecure and self doubting scarecrow in the story of The Wizard of Oz, I don't need a document or certificate from Harvard or some school of academic excellence to prove to myself that I have a brain. Often, these things are too overrated! But not only this, sometimes being systematically programmed or

---

[49] I think that the primary reason why I didn't get the job promotion was because others wanted to take the credit for another man's work.

brainwashed by a program of useless, academic material, which many universities and schools often disseminate, and that have no practical application in the real world, can be a waste of valuable time and assets. Also, I believe that sometimes, it can even stymie one's personal development, growth, advancement, and creativity in certain ways. Because often a person isn't encouraged to think for themselves. When you think about it, that may be one of the reasons why there hasn't been any outstanding discoveries and achievements in the world in recent years, like there was in the distant past. And why originally and creativity in many of the major fields of the arts, sciences, and so forth, has been pretty much drying up.[50]

Interestingly, Abraham Lincoln, Thomas Edison, Albert Einstein, and other great pioneers of progress of the past (people who did not have extensive formal educations), were not bogged down and inhibited by schools of higher learning. But, instead, they had the true freedom and liberty to sit and think deeply, to thoroughly explore the vast and exciting world and universe around them—to reach for the stars!

Sad to say, today, acquired personal knowledge, apart from formal education, is often not enough or valued as greatly by some. Instead, a person is required to have certain academic credentials and certificates to be taken seriously, or to get a job, etc.

Unlike the past, when a person was hired, and then conveniently trained on the job, today, it is often difficult to find and get decent employment without some type of certificate or degree. The crazy thing is, even when you spend the money, and put in the time to acquire these things, it doesn't necessarily guarantee that you're going to get hired in your field of study or interest, nor does it automatically guarantee advancement, good

---

[50] I'm not implying that schools of higher learning are completely useless. Because, to many this is what really matters in the real world. And sometimes, you have to take full advantage of this. However, what I am saying is that one's formal education does not necessarily determine a person's true value or worth.

wages, or success. And what's even more ironic about all of this is the fact that after you have gone through years of schooling and acquired all of the fancy degrees and certificates, you still have to be trained on the job! But, not only this, you're also left with a huge school loan debt that you most likely will have to spend the rest of your life paying off.

Making it a prerequisite for everyone to have or obtain an academic degree or certificate of some kind, in order to acquire gainful employment, is something that has been implemented in the field of employment only in recent years. Unfortunately, this makes it a whole lot harder on many, because everyone cannot afford the high price of education.

Personally, I think one of the major reasons why academic degrees, etc., have become prerequisites for many jobs in general, is because it is an intentional ploy to keep out and make it more difficult for the destitute, poor, and minority population to advance and succeed, especially with the passing of the Civil Rights Act of 1964, which outlawed employment discrimination based on race, color, religion, sex, and national origin. In essence, by making it a ruling or requirement to have proper academic credentials, it takes the pressure off of big corporations and businesses. Because, instead of them being forced to abide by fair hiring practices, it shifts the blame and responsibility onto the individual to succeed.

Don't get me wrong. In no way, am I anti-education. I believe that education is extremely important! But, I also think that there are many valuable things in life that can't be taught or learned in schools. And, as I look back at the past, I believe that this is one of the reasons why my mind was able to grow, and why my educational development and (Intelligence Quotient) IQ level shocked my career counselor and the tests administrator, despite the fact that I was only a lowly meter reader. The amazing thing is, because of my job (meter reader), I had both the freedom and time to pursue studies and other areas of personal interest (a wide variety of things), that I otherwise might not have been able to do, hadn't it been for that special field of employment and circumstance.

I know that this may seem somewhat corny or unrealistic to some people, but the truth of the matter is, I owe my entire education to God. He taught me everything that I know. But not only that, he is the one that initially sparked my interest and lit a fire in me. Because if I hadn't taken an interest in spiritual things in my early twenties, I would not have developed a love for reading, writing, and learning, which were things that I was not interested in prior to that time. Also, with God being the creator of all things in the universe, he gave me, along with everyone else, a thinking and reasoning mind or brain—one that is highly capable of acquiring and putting to use an endless amount of knowledge and wisdom.

The unfortunate thing is, the world doesn't always put a high value on knowledge that one acquires on their own through personal reading and study. Jobs and companies prefer their employees to have special academic credentials, or at least the bare essentials, from schools or educational institutions. Interestingly, they won't tell you this, but, sometimes, personal experience and knowledge is more preferred by them, because then they can greedily exploit and take advantage of any experience, knowledge, and natural abilities that you may possess, for their own benefit and gain — which often serves as an out or excuse for them, so that they don't have to give you the credit or pay you the dollar amount that you're really worth and rightfully deserve.

As we have seen and learned from the above examples and information, knowledge is important; however, it is not all-powerful. Nevertheless, we as humans, have to do our best to acquire it, and then use it for whatever benefits or good it offers, and to the best of our ability. By means of it, we can learn valuable things about ourselves, life, the amazing world, and the vast universe beyond.

One valuable thing that I've learned is that, not all negative things that we may go through in life are necessarily bad for us. Sometimes, we can learn a lot from them. Also, to suffer lost, can bring great gains!

Another important thing that I've learned (unfortunately, the hard way), is that of being forgiving — the amazing quality of continuing to display love to others, even when we don't seem to get anything back in return. True, it can be extremely challenging and hard to forgive others for the wrongs that they commit against us. But, it is the course of true wisdom. One valuable reason why is because it is good for our emotional, mental, physical, and spiritual health. For stored up resentment and anger can eat us up, destroying our peace, joy, happiness, and any potential good that we may have in us. Another reason why, is because when we practice forgiving it sets a good example for others, including our family and children (if we happen to have any).

Chapter 6

MARRIAGE AND FAMILY LIFE

A s of June, 2019, my wife and I have been married for forty-one wonderful years. And, although, before I got married, I wasn't looking to do so, when I first met my wife, for me, it was love at first sight. She was like an angel — the most beautiful girl I had ever seen! At the time, I thought to myself: *"Wow... that's the girl I'm going to marry!"* Although, of course, it wasn't that easy, for I had to later convince her of that. Luckily, for me, she eventually accepted my proposal. And we got married about six months later.

Initially, before I met my wife, I was a little skeptical and afraid of the thought of marriage, because it never seemed to work out for my mother who had married a number of times. Sure, I felt that one day I would possibly get married, but not until later in life, perhaps when I was in my mid thirties or so. Funny, it's strange how things sometimes turn out in life, and often a whole lot better than we would have anticipated or imagined!

My wife and I married in the year 1978. I was 22 years old at the time, and she was a couple of years younger. Eventually, we had three beautiful children, which led to having ten amazing grandchildren.

I love my kids, and when they were growing up, especially when they were young, I did a lot of things with them. We spent a lot of time at parks and lakes within the local area where we lived in the State of Minnesota — the land of 10,000 lakes. We also went on bike rides; we visited local zoos, theme parks, art and kid museums; we went shopping, and to the movies, and many other things. We also regularly took annual vacations in Florida. Some of the places we visited there were: the cities of St. Petersburg, Clearwater, Cocoa Beach, Orlando, and New Smyrna Beach. We also took the kids to Disney World, Sea World, Bush Gardens, and Universal Studios, etc. We always had a blast! — A fun filled, great time!

Not all Fun and Games

Although we had a pretty good and happy family life, the truth is, not everything was all fun and games. For instance, in the year 2000, my wife's body temperature for some unexplained reason began to run hot. Not knowing what the problem was, to combat this, she would eat a steady dose of ice chips. I was a little concerned as to what was causing her body to overheat, and why she had a craving for ice, so I suggested that she make an appointment to see our family doctor ASAP.

Later, when my wife was at her appointment at the doctor's office; during her medical examination, to her surprise, the doctor said that she thinks that she is having problems with her kidneys. And so she recommended that she see a kidney doctor, who is a kidney specialist.

After scheduling and visiting the kidney specialist, he recommended and arranged for a kidney biopsy to be performed on my wife. And, after the biopsy was completed, we were told that a sample of the tissue will be shipped to the lab, and that it takes about two weeks or so for the results to be completed.

Following the kidney biopsy, after two weeks or so went by; my wife received a phone call from the kidney specialist's office, who informed her that her test results are in. Also, they scheduled for her to come into the office, so that the doctor could let her know what the findings were.

A couple of days later, on the day that my wife went to her appointment at kidney doctor's office, I accompanied her there, just as I did on the day when she had the biopsy done.

Prior to this follow up visit with the kidney specialist, my wife and I had absolutely no clue as to what her test results would be, or as to what kind of news we would receive from the doctor. Unfortunately, to our dismay, shock, and disbelief, as it turned out, my wife was informed by the doctor that she has (immunoglobulin) Iga Nephropathy, which is an incurable, life ending kidney disease. What a gut wrenching, and devastatingly blow this turned out to be! Never in our wildest thoughts or dreams would we have ever imagined or expected to hear this kind of news! What an absolute shock, nightmare, and tragedy!

After absorbing this tremendous shock, and pulling ourselves together the best that we possibly could, the kidney specialist recommended that my wife immediately begin medical treatment, which involved close monitoring of her medical condition, and some other things.

Although it was an extremely difficult thing to ask, I asked the doctor how long my wife could live without medical treatment. He said: "Roughly speaking, about five years." Wow, what a complete and utter shock! To my wife and me, it was already too difficult to fathom or understand that she would ever have such a horrible illness like this, let alone to learn that her life could end so soon, and at such a young age!

The strange thing about all of this is, outwardly, my wife

seemed to be in perfectly good, physical health. Looking at her, you would have never even thought or imagined that she was sick or that she had a serious medical condition, in any form or way. As a matter of fact, up until the biopsy, we had absolutely no clue that she was ill! Apparently, one of the reasons why it's so hard to tell, is because, as they say, kidney disease is a silent disease or killer. And that it is not uncommon for it to lay dormant or go unnoticed in a person for years. As a matter of fact, it can go completely undetected until only about 10 percent of a person's kidney function is left. But then, that's when it's too late, when the wheels start coming off, so-to-speak.

At the time, because it was so difficult for my wife and me to believe and accept that she had a kidney disease; we decided to get a second opinion. So we schedule for this to be done at the world famous and prestigious, Mayo Clinic, in Rochester, Minnesota. However, to our disappointment, the second medical opinion only confirmed the first diagnoses to be thoroughly accurate and true. Afterwards, my wife immediately started medical treatment, which involved being closely monitored throughout the upcoming years by her kidney doctor, the one who first discovered and diagnosed her illness.

Unfortunately, as time passed; about six years after being diagnosed with the illness, in the year 2006, my wife's kidney disease progressed to End Stage Renal Disease (ESRD), which led to her experiencing complete renal failure, along with congestive heart failure.[51] Apparently, the reason why she suffered heart failure, along with renal failure, is because her lungs had filled up with fluid, because her kidneys were no longer functioning to remove it (a process that healthy kidneys regularly perform), so it all backed up into her lungs. As a result, this made it very hard for her to breathe, which put too much strain and pressure on her heart. This was a very scary ordeal! As a matter of fact, she almost died! Afterwards, she was immediately placed on kidney dialysis.

---

[51] End Stage Renal Disease is a medical condition in which a person's kidneys cease to function, leading to them needing long-term dialysis or a kidney transplant to maintain life.

Interestingly, the time frame of my wife's kidney failure was very close to her kidney doctor's prior prediction that he made in the year 2000. At that time he predicted that her kidneys would fail within about 5 years. So he was pretty accurate.

Initially, at the beginning of my wife's kidney dialysis, she started out receiving hemodialysis at a local kidney dialysis center — a process that took about four to five hours per treatment, being administered three times a week, on Mondays, Wednesdays, and Fridays. As it turned out, in the process, I used up a lot of my vacation days, and also took several leaves of absence from work. But if I had to, I'd do it all again. Because I was willing to do anything and everything to encourage and support my wife during this most discouraging and stressful time.

Sometime later, in the year 2007, my wife was informed that she is a good candidate for Peritoneal Dialysis (PD), which is a different type of dialysis for cleansing the blood and body of waste products. Interestingly, PD is a medical treatment that is conveniently administered or performed at one's home. This was a good thing, because peritoneal dialysis is a much better and cleaner process than hemodialysis. But also, it was better, because my wife would no longer have to travel to and sit at a depressing clinic. Instead, she would be receiving treatment in the privacy and comforts of her own home.

After agreeing to it, my wife was taken off hemodialysis ASAP, and placed on peritoneal dialysis. This required her to hook up to a kidney dialysis machine called a "Cycler" (that involved a very specific and detailed oriented, step-by-step, setup procedure, which takes a considerable amount of time to setup per treatment; each and every night, during bedtime). And she had to stay hooked up to this machine all night, until about 9 or 10 am the next day. The crazy thing is, she had to do this every night, nonstop, 7 days a week, 365 days a year, for the rest of her life, or until a possible kidney donor became available. Can you imagine how difficult that was for her to have to do this? Nevertheless, because of being the real trouper that she is, she thoroughly complied with everything that she was told and required to do. She simply had no choice, if she wanted to stay alive!

Only the Beginning of Woes

Unfortunately, my wife's kidney issues weren't the only problems that we had to face and deal with. Sad to say, in December of 2007, my eldest brother, Bernard, who was a singer, songwriter, and musician, committed suicide.[52] At the time he was sixty one years old. His death was a complete shock — totally unexpected! It hit our family like a ton of bricks! What a tragedy!

As far as life goes, none of us really know how it's going to turn out, or what it's going to bring us next. When I was growing up as a kid, I remember my Mom used to say: "When it rains, it pours!" And now, with all of the current problems and tragedies that we were facing, I would have to totally agree with her. But I never would have imagined the things that were to come next.

Unfortunately, later, in the year 2009, about two years after my wife experienced complete kidney failure, along with congestive heart failure; she fell and broke her hip, which was excruciatingly painful! This of course required immediate surgery. I stayed by her side the entire time while she was in the hospital.

Because I love my wife dearly, it was very difficult for me to have to see her suffer! I couldn't help but to think: *The poor thing, she's already been through too much as it is, having both kidney and heart issues, and now this!*" However, for her sake, I felt that I had to remain strong and be completely supportive. And, although it was emotionally hard on me, I did my best to try to conceal my feelings in front of her, so that it would not be discouraging to her.

Interestingly, the doctor who examined and operated on my wife's hip, said that the hip fracture most likely happened due to the prescribed medications that she was on; and also from being on

---

[52] The name has been changed.

peritoneal dialysis; both of which are notoriously known for thinning out the bones, making patients more susceptible to breakage.

Later, after about six months went by, my wife seemed to be recovering fairly well from her broken hip. But then, just when we thought that the storm of problems was coming to an end, and that sunshine was about to appear on the horizon, she was diagnosed with another problem. As it turned out, she was informed by her doctor that she has breast cancer. Oh no! Another huge blow! We were completely devastated! I felt so sorry and bad for my wife! I thought to myself: *"What else does this poor lady have to go through, hasn't she already suffered enough as it is?!"*

Immediately, my wife's cancer doctor prescribed and performed a lumpectomy, which was followed by aggressive radiation treatments. The good thing is that the cancer was caught in its early stage, and that during surgery they got or removed it all. However, the bad thing was, she was taken off the kidney donor recipient list. She was also put on cancer medications for the next five years, and told that she cannot be placed back on the kidney list until after she has proven to be cancer free for the next five years. This was more bad news that was just too hard to swallow! After all, five years is a very long time! Anything can happen during that time. Because of this, my wife and I wondered if she would ever recover and be healthy enough to be placed back on the list to receive a kidney transplant. Only time would tell!

Additional Storm Clouds

In the year 2010, just when we thought we were finally coming out of the woods, and that my wife's health was now starting to stabilize, another tragedy struck. My wife broke her other hip! As it turned out, this was only about one year later, after she had broken her first hip.

To add to the problem, while my wife was in the hospital being prep for hip surgery (this second time), her cancer doctor stopped in for a visit. And she informed us that the reason why she felt that my wife broke her hip was because she believes that her breast cancer has metastasized or spread to other parts of her body. And that she has progressed to Stage 4 cancer.[53] Wow, what a gut wrenching blow! What next, we thought?

Quickly reasoning upon what the doctor said, I told the doctor that it didn't make sense to me that my wife's breast cancer had metastasized; which was a response that the doctor didn't like. As a matter of fact, she got pretty upset with me, especially for what I told her next. I said to her: "How could my wife's cancer have metastasized, when the surgeons who performed the lumpectomy, assured us that they had gotten all of the cancer at that time. They also informed us that no cancer showed up or was found in her limp nodes."

I went on to further explain to my wife's doctor, saying: "The limp nodes are the human body's natural draining system. If my wife still had cancer after the lumpectomy was performed, it would have shown up when they examined the limp nodes at that time. But it didn't." In response, the doctor said nothing. Afterwards, she left.

After the doctor was gone, I tried to calm my wife's worries and fears, by telling her that I think that the cancer doctor is totally wrong! And that I don't believe that she has Stage 4 cancer! And that she's going to be ok!

Well, because of my insistence and refusal to accept the thought that my wife's hip fracture was the result of possible Stage 4 cancer, the prescribed medical plan or procedure set forth by her doctor and surgeon included; that during her surgery, the surgeon would remove a small portion of her hip bone, and then send it to the lab to have it analyzed for cancer.

Sometime later, after my wife's hip surgery had been

---

[53] There are 4 stages of cancer, with 1 being small, and 4 being large and more severe.

completed and she was in recovery, we were informed by the surgeon that operated on her that the operation was a complete success! He also told us that her lab results had come back, and that they showed that my wife's breast cancer did not metastasize. That she did not have Stage 4 cancer. This was a tremendous relief! We were very happy!

As you can see from this situation, that sometimes, it's best to take the bull by the horns so to speak, and become your own health advocate. If we hadn't done that, you never know what might have transpired. But not only this, by me having and maintaining a positive and optimist attitude and viewpoint, it proved to be of great comfort and support to my wife, to her spirit and mindset; especially, with her having to undergo surgery, not knowing what the final outcome might be.

A Double Whammy

With my wife having undergone so many health issues over such a relatively short period of time, I never even gave thought to my own personal health. Sure, I was suffering from some depression, but I never would have imagined what was to follow or come next.

Unexpectedly, in the year of 2010-11, I experienced a nervous breakdown. This was the day that I had spoken about earlier, in the Introduction of this book; the day when I was undergoing a panic attack, along with a psychotic episode. Unfortunately, in regards to the number of people having medical issues or problems in our immediate family, this was a double whammy, seeing that my wife already had her health issues.

I recall, on that most memorable day (the day when I suffered my breakdown), that I was scheduled to take my wife to the hospital. The reason why, is because she was suffering from a case of an iron deficiency, and she was scheduled to have an iron IV administered there. Apparently, iron deficiencies is one of the negative symptoms or effects of being on peritoneal dialysis, which can deplete a person's body of iron, as well as other necessary minerals and vitamins.

Unfortunately, the night before we left for the hospital, I was feeling a tremendous amount of stress. As a matter of fact, up until that time, I had never in my entire life been so stressed out before! The reason why is because I was undergoing a lot of strain and pressure at work for having recently exposed our company (a so-called reputable corporation) for failing to properly have some of their electronic test equipment, and other things (a significant number of items), which they were using to build life saving cardiac pacemakers and defibrillators, properly registered with the FDA.[54]

In addition to this problem, my wife and I had also recently lost our house due to foreclosure. Subsequently, this was a sad and distressing situation, to say the least, but at the time there was nothing that we could do about it. Although, I was working extremely hard for a promotion and pay raise at work, it just wasn't happening. Also, because my wife was disabled, and not capable of getting and working a regular job, there just was not enough money coming in.

~

The next day, when I woke up in the morning to drive my wife to the hospital for her medical treatment (to have the iron IV), I was feeling a little ill. I don't know what it was or what I might have caught. All I know is that I was feeling unusually strange — a feeling that I have never had before in my entire life.

My wife suggested that I take a shower. She said that it would probably make me feel better. So I took her advice and did what she said.

After showering, it seemed to help a bit. But I was still feeling somewhat strange and a little weird. So rather than driving, I had

---

[54] At the time I alerted only management of the problem. I didn't report these errors or problems out of spite or anything; I was just doing my job.

my wife drive to the hospital instead, while I sat in the passenger seat, along with our five year old granddaughter whom we happened to babysitting at the time.

A short time later, after finally arriving at the hospital, I was beginning to feel worse, so I had my wife drop me off at the front door, while she parked the car.

~

I was feeling all too strange, as I walked through the revolving glass doors at the hospital. I felt as though my mind was going to completely slip away from me! As I slowly moved through the doorway and into the lobby, suddenly, I felt like I just couldn't go any further, and that I needed to sit down. Luckily, there happened to be some chairs stationed there a short distance away from and directly facing the front door. So I immediately walked over and I took a seat.

Oddly and inexplicably, as I sat at the chair, I proceeded to glance back at the doorway. And when I did, I saw a most horrific sight! There were two women coming through the revolving door. The shocking thing is, the completion of their skin was chalky-white! the whitest white I have even seen! They looked like ghosts! And they had no eyes! but instead, in the socket areas where their eyes should be, there was large, round holes, that were pitch-black! Like charcoal. As the women passed by, they turned and they stared directly at me. What a frightening sight!

After the women left the area, I once again looked back at the front doorway. And when I did, I saw two paramedics wheeling a dead man on a gurney. They were entering the hospital through a standard doorway that is located right next to the revolving door. The weird thing is the dead man's body was lying uncovered and positioned in an upright sitting position of about a 45° angle on the stretcher.

As the paramedics wheeled the dead man pass me, I thought to myself: *"Wow... that sure is a strange sight! Why in the world are they bringing him through the front door and lobby of the hospital? This isn't the emergency room! But not only that, the guy is dead!"*

Suddenly, turning to my right, I looked, and I saw a doctor walking and moving towards me in slow-motion. He was fully dressed in blue surgical scrubs, with a cap on his head. And he was wearing protective booties over his shoes. As he passed by, he slowly turned and he looked straight at me. And then he gave me a very weird and chilling, eerie smile! I thought to myself: *"Oh no! It finally happened! — I think I lost my mind!"* And then, immediately, I began to feel extremely suspicious. For some reason, I felt that everyone there, within the vicinity of the hospital, knew that I had gone crazy, and that they were just waiting for me to outwardly show it, so that they could grab me, and quickly whisk me away to a nuthouse or something.

Panicking, I immediately got up and left the area where I was sitting. And I entered a men's bathroom nearby, so that I could hide. Moving quickly, I entered the bathroom stall, and I sat down on the toilet, but with my pants still pulled up. I actually didn't have to use the bathroom. I was just there to hide. Because I didn't want to get caught by anyone that I felt might be looking to find and get me!

Initially, when I first entered the bathroom, there was no one in there except for me. But then, suddenly, two men came in, which only served to heighten my fear!

Although I couldn't see who the men were, I could hear them whispering something to one another. However, I couldn't make out what they were actually saying. The bizarre thing is; and I don't know how I knew this (because I couldn't see them from where I was hiding), but one of them was a white man, and the other one was black. Still feeling paranoid, and not knowing what to expect, I sat there motionless and in silence, and then they eventually left.

After the two men were gone, I promptly got up and exited the bathroom. And then I walked over to and sat back down in the exact, same chair that I was initially sitting at when I first arrived at the hospital. I needed to sit down, because I was not feeling well.

As I sat there in the chair, a large and steady stream of people began to pass by. And then, suddenly, my wife appeared with our five year old granddaughter. But for some reason they didn't bother to stop or say anything to me. They just continued walking pass me.

The strange thing is that when my wife walked by, she turned and she looked at me, but then she quickly turned away. In response to her reaction, I thought to myself: *"Why is she ignoring me? Could it be that she realizes that I've gone crazy, and now she is afraid to be near me?"* Whatever the case, I felt that this was proof or confirmation that I did in fact, lose my mind.

I was both frightened and confused! I didn't know what to do! So I just continued to sit there in the chair for a moment. But then, afterwards, I quickly got up, and I followed after my wife and granddaughter, who were still walking and getting further away... Luckily, after having lost sight of them for a moment; looking up and into the distance, I was able to regain sight of them. They were entering an elevator. But by the time I got there, I missed it. So I waited for the next one to come.

As I waited at the elevator door, a small group of people who were traveling together, approached and stood by me. And when I turned and looked at them, I was completely shocked and taken aback! The reason being is because all of their faces were freakishly distorted and scary! So I quickly moved away from them and left the area. But, as soon as I walked away, I immediately got caught up in the flow of a large group of people who were walking through the hospital. And because they were pushing and pressing against me, I just went along with them, moving with the flow of the crowd. What a rush! I felt like I was floating down a river... being helplessly swept away by a raging torrent!

As I sheepishly and subjectively moved with the flow of the

fast and moving crowd, I became increasingly nervous and frightened, thinking that I was going to end up being pushed along and into an area or place where I didn't want to go. But, most importantly, I was getting too far away from where I needed to be, which was upstairs on the second floor with my wife and granddaughter.

Suddenly, the moving crowd that I was in, happened to pass by an in-house café and coffee shop. So I quickly mustered up the courage and strength that I needed to push my way out of the flowing herd of people. And I jumped in the food service line of a long and growing line of customers who were waiting to be served at the restaurant.

As I stood there waiting in the long, food line, it gradually got smaller and smaller, until finally it was my turn to be served. Subsequently, the restaurant's service counter girl, a young lady, smiled and looked at me, and said: "What can I get for you, Sir?" In answer, I said: "A cup of coffee please." Afterwards, I paid her; took the coffee; and then I walked over to and sat down at one of the café tables nearby.

As I sat there at the table, I was becoming increasingly frightened, paranoid, and confused! I didn't know what to do! I sensed that I was in a lot of trouble! But I was just too afraid to show or give any type of hint or sign to anyone that I had gone crazy or mad. Because I was fearful that if someone was to find out, that they would come and take me away and lock me up in a madhouse.

Sitting there, I tried my best to look like I was ok and normal, so as to blend in with everyone else. I attempted to take a drink of my coffee, but my hand was shaking so uncontrollably, that the coffee started to spill out of the cup. So I placed it back down on the table.

Suddenly, my legs started to grow numb, cold, and weak. Initially, the numbness began in my feet only, but then, it slowly and gradually started working its way up my legs. I was not feeling well at all! The truth is, I was in desperate need of help! But yet, I was too afraid to ask for it! What a dilemma!

As I sat there, people (other customers) began congregating all around me. Some were sitting at tables nearby, and others were coming and going. One person was a doctor, dressed partly in surgical scrubs and civilian clothes, who proceeded to walk over to and help himself to some condiments at the coffee shop condiment station nearby.

Because I was feeling both paranoid and afraid, I didn't know who to trust! Finally, after I remained sitting for a while, a middle-aged woman walked by me. And because I now realized that I could no longer put it off and that I was in desperate and immediate need of help, I finally mustered up the courage to ask her for assistance. I simply had no other choice! Because I was feeling all too strange, and the numbness in my body was only growing and getting much worse!

Getting her attention, I said to the woman: "Excuse me, Ma'am. But, I'm not feeling well!"

"What's the matter? Do you have the flu?" the Lady asked.

In response, I didn't know what to say. And I surely didn't want to tell her the truth — that I had simply gone mad! So I said: "Yep."

"Do you need a wheelchair?" She asked.

"Yes," I replied. And then she quickly turned and left.

After the woman left, within a moment or so later, two men, who were hospital staff workers or volunteers or something, approach me with a wheelchair. In response, I said to them: "I don't feel well!" So they kindly assisted and helped me get into the wheelchair.

While I was being seated in the wheelchair, I could hear one of the female workers at the restaurant service counter say to her fellow coworker, concerning me: "Ooh, girl! I told you not to be giving coffee to just anybody!" Afterwards, I was quickly whisked away by the two men.

As I was being wheeled down a long hallway, I gave the two men my full name and address. I also told them the reason why I was at the hospital — that I was there with my wife and granddaughter. And that my wife is presently upstairs on the second floor, being given an iron infusion treatment, because her body is low of iron. The men didn't ask for or request this information from me. I just voluntary gave it to them. Because I wanted to project an image that my brain was still functioning properly, and that I was mentally sound, so as to try to convince or fool them into thinking that I didn't really lose my mind after all, when in fact I did. Afterwards, I was quickly taken to the emergency room.

As I was being brought into the emergency room, I remember I felt like I was literally going to die. The reason being is that the cold and numb feeling that initially was in my feet, was steadily climbing and moving up my legs and body. Because of this I reasoned that once it reaches my heart, I'll be dead!

After the doctor and nurses in the emergency room quickly obtained information from me and examined me, they hooked me up to an IV (Intravenous Therapy), with appropriate medication. And they assured me that I was not going to die, but instead, that I was just having a panic attack.

"A panic attack?" I skeptically thought and quietly whispered to myself in disbelief.

Although I had never had a panic attack before, to me, what I was experiencing seemed to be a whole lot worse than a mere panic attack.

Later, I learned that it is not uncommon for one who is experiencing a panic attack to feel like they're going to die. This is often one of the symptoms.

As I laid there in the hospital bed, I started to weep and cry. I told the nurses that I feel so bad for my wife, because she has so many serious medical problems. I said that she has End Stage Renal Disease; heart issues; that she is a surviving cancer patient; and that she also broke both hips. And now, here I am dying and leaving her all alone! Again, the nurses comforted and reassured me that everything is ok, and that I was going to be alright.

Suddenly, in the background, I heard a woman screaming! She was another hospital patient who happened to be located in a separate and different room that was nearby. Frantically yelling and screaming, she said: "Let me go! I want my husband! Get my husband! He'll tell you to let me go!" Apparently, the lady was a mental health patient who was having some serious issues. As a matter of fact, I had overheard that she was being moved as soon as possible to the hospital's psychiatric ward. Thinking and reflecting on this, as I laid there in bed, I thought to myself that perhaps I was going to be the next one to also be taken there, having suffered a panic attack (along with experiencing a psychotic episode as I was later informed). But to me it really didn't matter, because I felt that I had lost my mind, and that I was in desperate need of help.

After some time had passed, and the effects of the medication gradually started to kick in, I started to calm down and feel much better. And then, surprising, both my wife and granddaughter arrived and entered the room.

"How did you know where I was?" I asked my wife.

"I heard about what happened," She said.

Apparently, the information that I provided the two men who wheeled me to the emergency room helped them to locate my wife and granddaughter, so that they could find them; explain to them what was going on; and let them know where I am. Luckily, shortly after this, I was released from the hospital, and my wife took me home. However, from that day forward, I was never the same again.

Interestingly, after experiencing a mental breakdown, it left me feeling mentally paralyzed and disabled to a large degree. Mentally, I felt like I had reverted back to my childhood. It was as though I had to start out all over again, learning from the beginning. When I think back as to why this occurred, I can now somewhat understand. I think the reason why this happened is because, even though the human mind is an amazing thing that is highly resilient and extremely adaptable, in reality it can only take so much pain and abuse. And after awhile, due to an extreme overload of suffering and pain, it shuts down to protect itself, in order to avoid further trauma, damage, and pain.

The fact is, I have experienced and gone through many things throughout my life, both good and bad. However, in my case, the bad or negative things that I experienced clearly overshadowed and outweighed the good. And as time progressed, the buildup of all of these things together became so heavy and great a weight, until the last situation or problem became the straw that broke the camel's back so to speak.

When it comes to the human body and brain, some things are just too complicated or difficult to be understood or explained. However, essentially, in my case, I believe that the area of the brain that controls emotions was broken or damaged — that perhaps a severance or break or some type of damage occurred within the connection between the thinking mind, and the heart (the seat of human emotion); and that my body did this in order to protect itself from any further or additional suffering and pain. In other words, the many negative things that I experienced in life, coupled with the final traumatic emotional experience that I suffered when I was working for the Pacemaker and Defibrillator Company (mentioned in chapter six of this book), caused serious damages to my brain's regulatory system; in particular, the area that regulates emotions — hence manic depression or bipolar disorder. The end result is that my brain no longer regulates emotions such as joy, sadness, etc., in the way that or to the degree that a "normal," healthy person might function or feel. It's not that I don't feel and display a certain measure of these things. It's just that my brain can no longer regulate the proper level or degree of these things that an emotionally and mentally healthy person might experience or feel in life. Can this be repaired or cured? Only time will tell.

When it comes to bipolar disorder; I personally think and believe that it is sometimes caused, not by just one thing alone, but rather through several or many different things all working together in unison — underlying issues or problems that we either knowingly or unknowingly experience and go though in life — things that gradually and progressively build up or accumulate over an extended period of time. Subsequently, the end result can be that the crushing weight from all of these weighty things together, winds up taking its toll upon a person's mind and emotions, and they eventually snap from the sheer force of the heavy burden and weight. It's like placing too much weight on a bridge — the overwhelming, heavy load can cause it to suffer a severe structural collapse. True, the human mind can be amazingly resilient and extremely strong in many ways. And it can often withstand a lot of suffering and pain. And yet, at the same time, it can also be very fragile too!

Personally, having been a victim of the "false image" of the "Negro," suffering from racial discrimination my entire life; being viewed and treated by white's as being inferior; being outcast by the black race in general; having to deal with many injustices and cruelties from both sides (the white and black race); coping with the death of my beloved mother, who was the mainstay and pillar of support in my life; having to deal with the serious illnesses affecting my beautiful wife; and finally, facing the possibility of being fired for being a whistleblower on the job; all of these things combined is a very heavy burden and load for anyone to have to carry, suffer, and bear. Consequently, as a result, I believed that the weight or burden from all of these things together are what eventually led up to me having a mental breakdown.

Interestingly, I would have to say that out of all of the things mentioned above, that the one thing that has been the most tormenting, troubling, and discouraging to me, is the unjust and discriminatory treatment that I have received throughout my life from a racist society that often undermines the true character, value, and beauty of its black and minority citizens.

A Shocking Revelation

Unfortunately, in the year 2010-11, I was diagnosed with bipolar disorder. At the time, I had become so withdrawn, and depressed, that eventually I was hospitalized for the purpose of having Electroconvulsive Therapy (ECT).[55] As a matter of fact, I was so bad off that prescribed medications and all other forms of therapy were just not working.

What I remember most about my time at the hospital, is that all that I talked about, over and over again, like a broken and skipping record, was how wrongly and badly I was treated by my managers at my place of employment — the Cardiac Pacemaker and Defibrillator Company. And how they hurt me, by failing to reward and promote me for the outstanding work that I did for them on the highly important and difficult projects that they gave me to do; all of which I had successfully completed to the companies great benefit... Pressing projects that no one else, including electronic engineers, and managers could not even come close to getting done.

Sometime later, during the ECT preparation process, my family and I, for personal reasons (based upon further information we received about the procedure, and its possible side effects), decided that it was best for me to forgo the treatment at that time. It's not

---

[55] Electroconvulsive Therapy (ECT) or Shock Treatment as it is sometimes referred to, is another treatment that can be used to treat bipolar patients. It is a procedure that is administered under general anesthesia, which involves intentionally feeding small currents of electricity into the brain for the purpose of inducing a brief seizure. Although, it is not fully understood how it works, it has been known to offer relief to some bipolar patients who suffer from debilitating depression.

that the treatment is bad or anything, it's just that it was not right for me at the time. Nevertheless, there are thousands of people yearly that have ECT treatments administered, and it has worked well for them. The good thing is that it's a personal discussion to decide whether to pursue this form of treatment or not.

Eventually, although I've gotten somewhat better (no longer feeling like a helpless child), to this day I still struggle to function normally on a daily basis. For the most part I am plagued with anxiety and depression.

As I suggested earlier in chapter two, I personally believe that environmental factor and influence played a significantly large role in my developing bipolar disorder, which is a theory that my life pretty much proves.

I believe in my situation or case that bipolar disorder is not due to genetics, but rather, that it began and developed over an extended period of time, through a series of stages, which were: (1) *bouts of depression,* (2) that gradually and progressively escalated to *chronic depression or mental illness,* (3) which in turn led to an *emotional trauma* that finally triggered *bipolar disorder.*

The fact is, over time, my depression was immensely fueled and greatly aggravated by an overly critical and negative environment or system of things that discriminates against blacks and minorities. And then, add to this, the problem of having to cope with the death of my beloved mother, and also coping with the serious illnesses affecting my beautiful wife, ending with a final emotional trauma that was brought on by my job — it was just too heavy of a load to carry and bear! The end result was a mental breakdown that triggered bipolar disorder.

Sunshine Appears on the Horizon

Five years after my wife was initially diagnosed and treated for breast cancer, we received some good news. We were informed by her doctors that she is now cancer free, and that she is being placed back on the kidney donor recipient list ASAP. This was wonderful news that made us very happy! Finally, some good news for a change! And it didn't stop there, for later, in the midyear of 2013, we received a phone call one late night, at about two o'clock am. It was my wife's kidney representative. She informed her that a donor kidney had just become available, and that they needed her to come to the hospital immediately, so that they can confirm that her and the kidney are a perfect match. However, the kidney representative made it perfectly clear that this was no guarantee that my wife would actually get the kidney, even if they were a perfect match. The reason being was that there were a couple of other kidney patients in line ahead of her to receive the kidney. They had first rights to it, seeing that they were higher up on the recipient list. But, just in case there was a problem with them failing to be a perfect match, my wife needed to be available and ready. To make a long story short, as it turned out, my wife was the only kidney patient out of the three that was a perfect match! We were absolutely thrilled!

Within the matter of a short time later, my wife had the kidney transplant, and everything has been going pretty well ever since. Sure, she's not perfect of course. But that's totally understandable and acceptable. Because, with her having been ill for so long (prior to having the transplant), obviously it had taken a toll on her overall health. Also, now that she had the transplant, her body is functioning on just one kidney alone (which the medical profession claims to be sufficient within itself), instead of functioning on two kidneys (something that is part of the normal, amazing, perfect design and structure of the human anatomy). Nevertheless, the good thing is, she no longer has to be on peritoneal dialysis; hooking up to a kidney dialysis machine every night, nonstop, 7 days a week, 365 days a year, which is something that she faithfully did for about seven years. What a blessing and relief!

Chapter 7

COPING WITH DEPRESSION

L ike many other illnesses, bipolar disorder or clinical depression is a disease, and those inflicted by it have no other recourse but to fight it, otherwise it can eat them alive. With this factor in mind, after a person is diagnosed with bipolar disorder, which initially can be a hard thing for them to personally accept; the first step in the battle, recovery, and coping process, is that they need to reach the point when they finally acknowledge and accept the fact that they actually have the illness, and that it is something that they most likely will have to deal and cope with the rest of their life.

Although being diagnosed with bipolar disorder can be a very difficult thing for one to accept, this is not something to be ashamed of, for it can happen to anybody. And with the right encouragement, support, and help, one can learn to successfully cope with the often debilitating disorder.

Fortunately, when it comes to dealing with bipolar disorder, there are many things that can help one to successfully cope — things that can comfort, encourage, refresh, and cheer a depressed soul. Things such as: being in a positive and uplifting social and home environment; having positive thinking and a healthy outlook; a good diet, and exercise; and receiving loving support and encouragement from family and friends. Also, in addition to these basic needs, there are many other things that one can choose to incorporate into, or eliminate from their lives that can help, which I will also briefly touch on in this chapter.[56]

Interestingly, when it comes to searching for, finding, or utilizing things that can help one to deal and cope with bipolar disorder, there is no one thing alone that will do the trick — like swallowing a magic pill or something. Instead, I personally find that it takes a combination of a number of things, all working together in unison. So let's us consider some of these things, one at a time.

A Positive Social Environment

When it comes to a person's emotional and mental health, a positive and uplifting social environment is vital for everyone. Not only is it an important factor in one's development and growth as an individual, but it is also good for their overall health and wellbeing too.

Positive environments are absolutely essential. The reason why is because they provide encouragement and support — the basic ingredients or things that all humans desire and need to feel secure, happy, appreciated, and loved. On the other hand, negative environments can be detrimental to one's overall health and wellbeing. Because they are often devoid of the love, encouragement, and support that humans need to be well rounded and happy individuals.

---

[56] Although prescribed medications can help people to cope with bipolar depression, I won't be touching on this particular method of treatment at this time.

All people need positive social environments, but especially is this absolutely necessary and essential for bipolar disorder patients who suffer from debilitating depression. Because it makes them feel better when they are around people who value them, treat them with love, understanding, dignity, kindness, and respect. On the other hand, overly critical and negative environments can create insecurities, sadness, and depression in people. But they can also further add to or feed one's bipolar depression, making matters a whole lot worse!

Unfortunately, when it comes to environments, most of us don't have much of a choice or say as to what kind we live in or grow up in. Often, we are left to make the most of a good or bad situation, depending on what it's like. However, in regards to some aspects concerning environments and our individual involvement in them, there are certain things that we do have the ability or power to improve or change, even if it's to a minimum degree — things that can have a significant and positive impact upon both ours and other peoples overall health and wellbeing.

An interesting thing is that social environments are a lot like people or personalities. In that each has its own distinct features or characteristics that make them unique and different from one another. Some are warm and inviting, others are cold and aloof, some are encouraging and supportive, while others are overly picky and critical, and so forth. And then, there are those that have a mixture of these things, and more. The social environments that I'm referring to are *long-term environments*, those that we spend a considerable amount of time in, such as at school, work, or in our neighborhood, etc.

When it comes to the overall makeup or structure of environments, it is often virtually impossible to significantly alter or change them, because their characteristics or personalities are generally already solidly fixed or set in stone. And because of this, the only three choices that people usually have are: (1) They can choose to stay within their environment, and adapt and become like it. Thereby contributing to its production and success, and sharing in its failures, and so forth, or (2) They can decide to remove themselves from it to avoid its effects and influences, or (3) They can hate it and complain about it, but decide to stay within it, and be unhappy and miserable.[57]

Interestingly, there are some environments that we fit into better than others. Also, what works for one person, may not be a good fit for another. The truth is no environment is perfect. And if it becomes necessary to choose one, it often comes down to selecting the one that suits us the best — one that we can at least tolerate and function within to a reasonable degree.

But, what if the environment that we find ourselves within is just too overly critical and negative, so much so that it is to the point of being damaging to us? What do we do then?

Avoiding overly critical and negative environments. Environments can be an important factor in regards to our personal peace, happiness, health, development, and growth. Often, they can make or break us, depending on whether they are supportive and encouraging, or unsupportive and discouraging.

Interestingly, it is not uncommon for people who suffer from bipolar disorder to have feelings of worthlessness or low self-esteem. And when they are in the company of people who view and treat them like they are insignificant, useless, or good-for-nothing, it only serves to intensify those negative feelings. Personally, I try to avoid *overly critical and negative* people, environments, or places that make me feel this way, because I find them to be counterproductive, discouraging, emotionally draining, and damaging. It's not that I think that I am better than others, because I'm not. It's just that I realize that there are certain things

---

[57] Sometimes there may be overly challenging, negative environments that we find ourselves in, because we have no other choice but to stay and try to function within them... because, due to one reason or another we cannot leave or remove ourselves from them, or we simply have no other place to go. (For help on how to develop, grow, and be productive in an over challenging and negative environment, see the information "Growing and Developing in a Negative Environment," in Appendix A, on page 244)

that feed my depression, making it worse. And it is best for me to steer clear of these for my own emotional health and wellbeing. The fact is, I'm already mentally beat-up and down as it is. I don't need to add to this, by allowing others to cause me further suffering and pain.[58] To see the bad and negative effects that criticism can have on a person, see the information "Constructive Criticism?" in Appendix A, on pages 242-243.

Having major depression is like continuously battling or wrestling with an unrelenting enemy — one who is bent on trying to tear you down and defeat you. Therefore, it's important for those who suffer from depression to never let down their guard. They must be ever vigilant to avoid situations, areas, things, and even certain people at times, that might feed their depression and cause them further mental and emotional pain.

In regards to people, most of us know what it's like to be around difficult individuals, such as a bully, or an overly rude person, or a person who is a killjoy — one who spoils, crushes, or kills any and everything that we say or do (even if they are positive and valuable things). These kinds of people are like damaging weeds that sprout up in a garden, and eventually overtake and choke the growth, vitality, and beauty from the healthy plants. Unfortunately, throughout history, these damaging weeds or individuals have taken their tow on many people, crushing and destroying their potential good, goals, and dreams.

Due to the excessive severity of some negative influences, and the bad and harmful effects that they may have on us personally,

---

[58] Notice that I said that I try to avoid *overly* critical and negative people and environments, not just critical or negative people and environments in general. The reason why is because negativity can be found everywhere. This is just a normal part of everyday life. And it is something that we must get used to dealing with. However, it is the extreme, *overly* critical and negative ones that put it over the top, which sometimes makes it very hard to cope and deal with. These are the ones that, because of my depression, and the environment's harmful effects on me, that I, if possible, personally try to avoid. Note: I'm not recommending this way of handling these kinds of situations or environments to others. It's just something that I find that I personally need to do at times.

sometimes, if possible, it may be necessary to avoid overly critical and negative environments that have a discouraging or detrimental effect on us. But then, in return, we need to replace these with positive ones that will be healthy for us emotionally, mentally, and physically — good environments, that will be helpful and supportive, and that will encourage us and uplift our spirits, especially in times of need.

But, what if it is not feasible for us to bodily remove ourselves from an overly negative and critical environment, because for one reason or another, we happen to be stuck there, with no other place to go? What might we do so that its harmful influence doesn't impact us too greatly? Well, one thing that can help is by having a realist view of life and people in general.

Having a realist view of life and people. Life is a beautiful thing, and there are a lot of wonderful and exciting things around us; things that make life enjoyable, but that we often take for granted. However, on the flipside of things, there are also negative things that we often have to face, cope, and contend with — challenging things that can sometimes make life tough and hard to deal with.

One thing that can make life difficult or challenging is that we have to daily navigate our way through a vast sea of people that possess a variety of likes, dislikes, attitudes, personalities, ambitions, life styles, and goals, etc.... that are often completely different from our own. And because of this, we must learn to accept variety or diversity. But we also have the challenge of staying true to ourselves, by not allowing the often highly opinionated, pushy, and domineering world around us squeeze us into its mold, which can cause us to lose sight of our own distinct individually — the special and unique characteristics that make us who we are.

In addition, the attitude or spirit of the world around us can be highly competitive. Many people are daily fighting for dominance in one thing or another, whether it is for attention, power, prominence, jobs, money, or material wealth, etc. These things are so important to some people that they will do anything to succeed or obtain them, even if it means stepping on as many heads and toes that they can, no matter who it is, as they scratch and claw their way to the top. Unfortunately, sometimes we unforeseeably get in the path of these overly aggressive and ambitious one's, and we become a victim of misfortune. And in the end, we are left there, lying hurt on the side of road, shaking or scratching our heads in utter disbelief, as we try to contemplate or piece together what had just happened, or what the person's problem is.

A strange thing is, although you wouldn't necessarily expect it to be this way (because naturally you think that they would try to be more like the one that they claim to worship and represent); one of the most challenging and negative environments to inhabit sometimes, can be a religious environment (no religion or denomination in particular). The reason being is that many of its enthusiasts are often too overly critical, negative, and suspicious of others. Perhaps, it is because they think that they are better than others due to their seeming or imagined favoritism or relationship with God. Or maybe they are afraid of being influenced or contaminated by the pagan or heathen or anything unholy. Whatever the case or their thinking may be, it has a tendency to make them not only cocky and arrogant, but also overly judgmental, negative, critical, and nitpicky about everyone and everything, even to the smallest of degrees.

Sad to say, their holier than thou disposition often makes them blind to their own faults and imperfections. And if you where to kindly and tactfully point this out to them, they would say that you are highly mistaken. And then, rather than putting forth the efforts to change for the better, they completely excuse themselves of any errors, and then they turn around and put the blame solely on you instead. Unfortunately, the problem is, like the self proclaimed holy man (the hypocrite), some are so busy examining everyone else and their shortcomings with a magnifying glass, that they fail to realize that *all* people, including themselves, are sinners, who are forever in need of God's undeserved kindness, mercy, and forgiveness. And that we need to focus mainly on ourselves, and not others. Because, in realty we don't have the power to change anyone, except for ourselves, and even this is only through the grace and help of God. Interestingly, some of the bloodiest wars in history have been fought in the name of religion.

I'm not insinuating or saying that being religious is a bad thing, because it's not. Neither I'm I saying that all religious people are overly negative and critical, because many of them are very beautiful, sincere, loving, helpful, and encouraging individuals. What I am saying is that negativity is found everywhere, and that sometimes we need to be cognizant of our environment, so that we don't fall into the trap of unknowingly allowing the personal viewpoints and thinking of certain people to discourage us and cause us unnecessary problems or pain.

Another challenging thing that can be hard to cope and deal with at times is human imperfections. The fact is none of us are perfect. And because of this, both we and others are going to say and do things at times that may hurt and offend one another. Knowing and understanding this can be very helpful, because if someone happens to hurt or offend us, which they inevitably will; we won't be too quick to get upset or take offence, allowing it to ruffle are feathers so-to-speak.

Another thing that can help is when we don't expect too much from others. But instead, we are willing to accept them for whom and what they are. I'm not saying that we should necessarily compromise our standards or beliefs. What I am saying is that it helps when we are not too demanding and overly critical of people. For if we have the habit of setting the bar too high in what we expect from others; we are sure to be disappointed. But on the other hand, if we allow for errors and imperfections in others, then we won't be too devastated or bent out of shape when they disappoint us.

Another thing that can help us to cope and fair well within an overly critical and negative environment, is when we are willing to forgive others for the hurt or harm that they cause us, whether it is done intentionally or unintentionally.

Practice forgiving. An old and wise familiar proverb says: "To err is human; to forgive is divine." Meaning that it is human nature to sin and make mistakes. And yet, God freely forgives us. And when we forgive others we are being like him.

Unfortunately, many of us are still harboring and battling things today that have happened to us in our youth or distant past. Highly disturbing and troubling things that left emotional scars that keep resurfacing and that don't seem to ever be going away. For example, sometimes we let others unduly influence how and what we think about ourselves. In effect, we let them plant negative thoughts and images in our mind — lying pictures and scenes that rob us of our internal peace, joy, and happiness. Images that make us hate ourselves, or that make us feel like we are ugly, inferior, failures, or losers.

What can help us to change, so that we no longer have to suffer from these things, and go on to lead happier, productive lives? The answer is to forgive, and then move on.

What does it mean to be forgiving? It means to *completely pardon* or let go of a wrong that a person committed against us. To cease from feeling resentment and anger towards them, and not wanting, desiring, or seeking retaliation or revenge.

Personally, in the past, where I went wrong in my life, was that I allowed the discriminatory and overly critical and negative environment around me, along with the hurtful experiences that I suffered at the hands of others, influence my thinking, and also dictate my self-worth, which led to a lot of crippling emotional pain and depression. Unfortunately, these hurtful things and experiences changed my viewpoint, focus, and thinking, from that of being wholesome and healthy, to being negative and critical of pretty much everyone and everything, including myself. But it also led to me not wanting to be around other people; out of fear that I would become a victim of their further cruel judgments, pranks, and remarks. As a result, I pretty much became a loner in life, which sometimes can serve as a protection, because it can shield us from additional pain. However, it can also be crippling to us too, because we can develop tolerance and valuable coping skills from being around other people.

Unfortunately, by letting the bad experiences that I had with people stumble me, it wound up stunting my emotional develop and growth to a certain degree. As a result, it kept me from gaining maturity and stability in certain aspects of my life. And it also robbed me of a certain amount of inner peace and joy. But not only that, I did not set a good example for others. Now, as I think back on these things, I realize that I would have been much better off, if I was forgiving and didn't take things so personal, allowing frustration and anger to take root and grow. Luckily, in time, I wised up and learned from my past mistakes.

Why is forgiving so important? Well, for one, we are all imperfect humans, who are in need of forgiveness. It is also important because there are good benefits that come to us when we both willingly and freely forgive others. For one, it helps us in our relationships and friendships with others. But it is also good for our overall health and wellbeing too. Because when we forgive and forget we don't have to carry around the heavy weight and burdens of feeling hurt, anger, resentment, and hatred; all of which are strong deterrents and barriers to our own inner peace, joy, and happiness. But also, being unforgiving can be harmful to our personal health. For living with bad feelings and emotions can make us ill.

The role feelings and emotions play. As humans, we were created with the ability to be able to express a wide range of feelings and emotions. We can express love, affection, joy, kindness, empathy, compassion, and the list goes on and on.

While feelings and emotions can add color and spice to our lives, making it more enjoyable; on the flipside of things, if we are not watchful and careful, certain *bad* feelings and emotions can do the exact opposite. They can bring us sorrow and pain. But even worse than this, they can be damaging to our health, because our deep feelings and emotions support our overall health and wellbeing—physically, mentally, and spiritually. Interestingly, human emotions can run so deep that people have been known to literally die from a broken heart. Also, fits of uncontrolled rage and anger can be damaging to one's health. They can cause high blood pressure, respiratory issues, digestive troubles, skin diseases, hives, ulcers, and a host of other health issues.

Personally, as regards myself, I think my bad feelings and emotions were one of the main causes of my clinical depression; negative emotions that were brought on and agitated from growing up and living within an overly critical and negative environment or society that unjustly discriminates against blacks and minorities; an environment or established system, which, today, has resulted from the "false image" that was handed down to the black race, that originally got its start during the time of institutional black slavery in America.

As we can see from the examples above, *bad* feelings and emotions can be detrimental to our health and overall wellbeing. However, on the other hand, *good* feelings and emotions can be good for our health. Interestingly, in the Bible at Proverbs 16:24 it tells us: "Pleasant sayings are a healing to the bones." (New World Translation) Meaning that positive and uplifting words of encouragement that we receive from others can have an uplifting affect on our moods and health. They can cheer us up and make us feel better.

Because bad feelings and emotions can run deep, sometimes it can be a real challenge to gain control over them, especially if we are experiencing or undergoing extremely difficult and trying situations. But, in spite of this, for one's own health and wellbeing, it is best to try to have and maintain a positive attitude and spirit. One way that we can be helped to do this is by having support and help from others who are interested in our wellbeing. However, not all associations are helpful in this regards, as a matter of fact, some may be the exact opposite. Instead of encouraging a positive attitude, they may promote a negative spirit and attitude in us. With this being the case, what might we do that can help us in this area?

Watch your associations. It's been said: "Show me who your friends are, and I'll tell you who you are." There is a lot of truth to this statement, because those with whom we choose to associate, we often become like.

In addition to having a powerful influence on us, people that we hang out with, can either build us up or tear us down. So depending on whether we wish to fair well or bad, it is important to choose our friends and associates wisely. This includes not only physical friendships, but also associates that we invite into our lives through the media, TV programs, and the internet, etc. These too are our associates. And they can ether have a positive or negative influence on us. To give you a personal example of this, in the past I use to ritually watch the daily news reports on TV. But, recently, I had to stop watching these because they made me feel sad and depressed, with all of the bad news that they daily featured and reported on.

Interestingly, within a short period of time, after I quit watching the daily news, I noticed that my thinking and outlook changed for the better. Because I was no longer allowing the sad, shocking, and disastrous things that were often being reported on to influence my moods in a negative way. Sure, occasionally, I'll catch something on the news here and there (concerning the weather or sports or something), but, for the most part, I try to avoid them altogether. Interestingly, it's sort of ironic when you think about it, but sometimes the less that we know or the less informed that we are, the better off we are. I know this to be true in this case, because I am no longer allowing the sad and discouraging news reports to feed my depression and pull me down.

From life's experience I have come to learn that there are certain situations, areas, and even particular people at times that can feed and breed depression in us. And that for our own health, wellbeing, and protection, we need to be ever cognizant or aware of what and who these might be. And, if it happens to be within our power and ability to control or change matters, then we need to take the appropriate actions or steps necessary to either minimize the negative effects and influences that these have on us personally, or to remove them entirely.

However, when it comes to shutting off associations with people, there is a certain caution that we need to be aware of, which is the trap of falling into complete and total isolation.

Avoiding total isolation. Although avoiding certain environments and people may be necessary from time to time, there is need for caution in this area. The fact is, it can only be done to a limited degree, for complete isolation can be damaging to us personally. The reason being is that by nature, we as humans were made to be social creatures. For the most part we need other people in our lives to communicate and socialize with, for this can be good, beneficial, and healthy for us. True, sometimes we need a little solitude; some quiet time alone, for this can have its benefits too. However, too much time alone is not good. So fight off the tendency or urge to want to lock yourself alone in your room. Although this may initially feel somewhat good, in the long run it can be crippling and damaging to us personally.

When it comes to life, although a bit of self sufficiency and self reliance has its place in the world, it is best not to try to go through life alone, but instead, to have and solicit support from family, friends, and others, who will encourage and uplift our spirits along the way. Interestingly, it doesn't have to be a large group. It could be just one or two people, who together with ourselves, make up a strong and supportive team. This is vitally important, because life can be hard, and there will be trying times when we need a little encouragement, direction, support, and help from others. In the Bible it says: "Two are better than one... for if they fall, the one will lift up his fellow: but woe to him that is alone when he falleth; for he hath not another to lift him up."—Ecclesiastes 4:9-10. (King James Version)

A Positive Attitude and Healthy Outlook

Cultivating a positive attitude and healthy outlook. Traveling on the ever changing and challenging road of life is much better when we cultivate a positive attitude. This can help the road to be a little smoother and easier to travel on. But it can also make the difference between either leading a peaceful, contented, and happy life, or living a miserable one.

I say to *cultivate* a positive attitude, because having a positive attitude is something that many of us have to regularly work hard at manifesting or displaying in our lives. The reason being is that it doesn't necessarily come easy. As a matter of fact, having and maintaining a positive attitude or healthy outlook can be one of the most difficult things that we can do in life. The reason being is because we already have the deck stacked against us so to speak, in that we are all imperfect creatures, and sometimes our own shortcomings, or those of others, can get us down. Also, there may be certain difficult situations that we may be facing, or overly negative and critical social environments that can be downright discouraging and challenging to us.

Another thing that can make having a positive attitude challenging, is having bad heath. For it can negatively affect one's thinking and outlook. Because, when we are suffering and in pain, it can be hard to focus on the positive aspect of things—to see and appreciate the good and beautiful things around us. To give you an example, I'll tell you a true story that happened to me. As it is, my wife and I live in the northern state of Minnesota. So we like to vacation during the cold winter months in sunny Clearwater, Florida; an annual three week trip in which we use to drive. Well, one year during our drive there, I suddenly developed a toothache. Initially, the pain was controllable through the use of a little aspirin. But, the further we drove, the greater the pain got. Finally, when we arrived at our destination, the pain was so intense that I had to seek emergency help from a local dentist, who started root canal work immediately on the bad tooth — a process, which at the time took three separate appointments. Well, after the first part of the dental procedure was done, the dentist set up the next appointment and then sent me on my way. Interestingly, the initial work that was done on my tooth seemed to help somewhat; that is until the Novocain wore off. Then, I was in excruciating pain all over again!

Now, sunny Clearwater, mind you, is very beautiful. The scenery is absolutely breathtaking, with its decorative palm trees, its delightful array of various blooming flowers, white sandy beaches, and crystal blue waters. However, because the pain that I was experiencing was so excruciating and unbearable, I could not see and appreciate the paradisiacal beauty that surrounded me. All I could focus on was the miserable and unbearable pain. So I returned to the dentist, but this time I decided to have the tooth, which was one of my back teeth, pulled instead. And, although I lost a valuable, irreplaceable tooth; what's amazing is that the moment the tooth was extracted, the pain immediately stopped. And now, finally, I could see, smell, feel, and appreciate all of the beauty of the tropical paradise that surrounded me — something that I could not appreciate when I was in pain. Well, the same can be true of those who suffer from an illness, such as clinical depression or bipolar disorder. Often, the emotional pain that one feels is so intense that it makes it very hard to focus on the good, beautiful, and positive things around them. However, it can be done, even if it is to a limited degree.[59] And for one's own wellbeing and health sake, it is both advantageous and vitally important that they continue to put forth an earnest effort to try. So, if you are having difficulty in this area, what are some things that you can do that might help you to be more positive?

Feeding the mind positive things. One of the best things that we can do for our mind or brain is to feed it valuable, good, positive, and uplifting things. This is vitally important to our emotional, mental, and physical health. Nevertheless, this is not always an easy thing to do. One reason why is due to human imperfection. Because we are all inherently imperfect and sinful, we have an

---

[59] Although I truly have hope and believe that God has a bright future in store for the earth and me, I often struggle with having a positive outlook. The reason why is because of bipolar disorder and its vicious cycle. In particular, the down or "depressive phase." The truth of the matter is, it can be very hard to cope during this period of time, when you're experiencing sad and dark moods. However, the good thing is that it will eventually pass (when the time for entering the "euphoric phase" comes), when you feel emotionally up and energetic. And because of this I try to exercise patience, and take comfort that the time is coming when I will be feeling better again.

inborn tendency to gravitate towards bad things. The degree to which we do this may vary, depending on each individual. Some may have a lesser or greater craving to feed their mind on negative things. For example, some people have the bad habit of being nitpickers or fault finders. Instead of looking for the good in things and others, they tend to focus on the imperfections and negative things. Some even take pride in being able to find and point out small imperfections or flaws in people or things that others don't seem to see or notice.

If we see ourselves being like this overly critical and negative person, then we need to stop doing this, because it is damaging to both ourselves and others. Life is better when we look for the good in people and things, not the bad. For some people this may not be easy, especially if we have a habit or long history of faultfinding and negative thinking, or if we suffer from depression. Because, when we're down and depressed it's so easy to gravitate towards the negative. However, if we put forth genuine and real effort, we can change and train our minds to think positive.

One thing that can help us to be positive is to think of ourselves as being a skilled artist or painter, and our minds as being a large canvas on which to paint. Now, in respects to our own personal canvas, we have the choice to create and paint whatever scene we want on it. So what colors and subjects would you choose to paint? No doubt you would choose warm and vibrant colors, and a most delightful and beautiful scene, especially if you intend on hanging your finished painting on the wall or in an area for you and all to see and enjoy. Well, the same can be true of our minds and what we allow or choose to feed and occupy it. We have the choice to fill it with whatever scenes and subject matter we want. Yes, we can make or create any kind of world that we wish on the ever changing and highly adaptable canvas of our mind. Luckily, for us, the world and creation around us is full of many wonderful, delightful, beautiful, exciting, and inspiring things to select from, so we don't have to travel or go too far to find them.

Unfortunately, for some people who suffer from an illness such as bipolar disorder, seeing and thinking positive may not be an easy thing to do. Because they are suffering from depression or experiencing emotional pain it may be harder for them to see and appreciate the beauty of things around them. However, they too, can be helped in this regards. True, it may take greater effort. But it can be done. So what can help?

As it so happens, the world is not short on garbage and junk food that we can figuratively feed on. It serves up a daily dose and endless supply of ignorance, violence, and other bad and negative things, which can be readily found by simply turning on the TV, by connecting to the internet, or playing certain video games, etc. So if we want to be positive and mentally healthy, we need to be *selective* in what we choose to watch and be influenced by. In this regards we need to search for good and positive things.

Searching for good and positive things. It's been said that we are what we eat. And, although this is not always or completely true in every respects, to a certain degree having a good physical diet can be beneficial to our health. Well, the same is true concerning what we choose to feed our minds.

Interestingly, it has been said that life is all about choices. So with regards to the matter of choices as to what we choose to consume and fill our minds with, what will you choose?

In regards to physical food, we often seem to crave and love to eat the things that may not be good for our health; things like fast-food, sweets, and junk foods. Sometimes we just can't get enough of them. But, for our own good and overall health we have to exercise restraint when it comes to these things. The same can be true when it comes to the mental food and diet of things that we feed our minds. Correspondingly, like physical food, our minds also often crave what is not good and healthy for us. But, just like fighting the craving to eat physical foods that are bad for our health, we have to get tuff with ourselves and fight the tendency to fill our minds with things that can be detrimental to having positive thinking and a good outlook on life. True, it's not that having a healthy mental diet is going to necessary cure us of our depression, but it can to a certain degree make our lives a whole lot better.

When it comes to the thought process, it is only natural to have negative thoughts from time to time, that's only part of being human. But the key is to not to allow ourselves to dwell on them, so that we are not overcome by them. Subsequently, in order to combat this, the best thing to do when we start to have negative thoughts is to immediately dismiss them and put them out of our mind. And then we need to key in and focus on things that are positive, good, and healthy for us instead.

No doubt about it, fighting to be and stay positive can be a very hard and challenging thing to do, but we have no choice if we want to succeed and be better off. The truth is, negative thinking feeds and fuels depression. It can be like being in quicksand. The more negative we are or become, the further we can sink deeper into the pit of misery and despair.

So if we are fighting to stay positive, what things might we focus on or consider? Well, in the Bible at Philippians 4:8 it says: "Whatever things are true, whatever things are of serious concern, whatever things are righteous, whatever things are chaste, whatever things are lovable, whatever things are well-spoken-of, whatever things are virtuous, and whatever things are praiseworthy, continue considering these things." Why? Because these things are not only good and healthy, but they also serve as a protection for us.

Sometimes, because positive things may not seem to be readily present or apparent, or they don't happen to jump out at us, we may have to make a diligent search to find them. The fact is, there are many beautiful, positive, and inspiring things all around us, but sometimes all we need to do is just take the time to be observant and look.

Find your joy. In observation, I've noticed that it is human tendency, that when a person is down, or they feel bad about themselves or something, that often they will look for, pursue, or do things that make them feel better. In particular, this seems to happen a lot with people who suffer from depression or some other type of mental or emotional pain. However, in a large percentage of these cases, one usually winds up gravitating towards things that make matters much worse, by filling or replacing the hurt or pain with alcohol, illicit drugs, binge eating, or some other harmful things. In the end, the person's misery or pain often becomes worse, because they are left with a bad addiction, or a troubling and guilty conscience, etc. If you happen to be one that this is happening to, why not try to find or pursue something that is good and healthy for you instead. In other words, find your true *joy* or passion in life — the one, positive, good, and healthy thing that will make you feel better about yourself and life; something that is going to add true value to your character, and that will build you up, rather than tear you down.

What might you choose? Well, it could be virtually anything; from becoming a gourmet chef, a photographer, a writer, an artist, such as a painter or sculpturist; a musician or learning to play an instrument; or simply deepening your relationship with God. Undoubtedly, there are many things to choose from. The choice is totally up to you. The point is to fill the void or hurt in your life with something that is good and beneficial, something that will bring you a true measure of peace, satisfaction, and happiness.

Keeping active. Another thing that can help us to stay positive is by keeping busy and active. It's been said that "An idle mind is the devil's playground." So, sometimes, in order to put or keep ourselves in a better frame of mind, we have to get up, move about, and keep active. Interestingly, I've often noticed that in observing senior citizens, that the ones that are usually the most joyful and healthy, are the ones that are always active and busy in one way or another.

Love and respect yourself. It is vitally important that we love and respect ourselves for whom and what we are. Not to the point of being a narcissist, but rather to a healthy or balanced degree. So get to know yourself and accept who you are as a distinct and wonderful individual. Unfortunately, it took me some 60 years of my life before I finally figured this out. Sadly, during the process, I lost a lot of valuable time, because I allowed other things to sidetrack and distract me. But now, I am thoroughly enjoying spending every remaining minute with the beautiful person that I found and discovered inside of me.

Unfortunately, the truth of the matter is, we often don't see or appreciate ourselves for who we are as a distinct and beautiful individual. Because we often allow the distorted views or negative opinions of others get in the way and influence us, which, in turn, often leads to a sort of self hatred and self destruction — resulting in the self infliction of beating ourselves up, both mentally and emotionally.

The truth is we can be our own worst enemy or critic. And, although it's good to examine and censure ourselves from time to time, the important thing is that we should never be too hard on ourselves, because this can lead to having a bruised or crushed spirit, which can cause and feed depression.

Sad to say, discontentment and self hate can rob us of so many good and valuable things in life. Things such as self discovery, which can help us to learn many interesting and amazing things about ourselves, including discovering innate abilities and gifts in us that we didn't even realize we possessed. It can also rob us of development and growth, and being able to experience to the greatest extent possible the inner qualities of peace, joy, and self love—good and healthy qualities and thinking that can add to our enjoyment and happiness in life. Because, by focusing on negative and self destructive things, we can stifle the growth of these things within us. But also, a self destructive attitude and spirit can also be damaging to our personal health—mentally, emotionally, physically, and also spiritually. So don't miss out on the good things of life by sabotaging your own personal wellbeing and happiness, by being too overly critical and negative about yourself.

What are some things that can help us to come to love, appreciate, and respect ourselves? Well, for one, I find that it is best when we don't live and judge ourselves by other people's opinions, standards, and ways. The fact is, no matter how hard we try, we will never be able to please everyone. Another thing is, don't make the mistake of comparing yourself to others, because everybody is unique and different. Other people have their abilities and strengths, and we have ours. Also, learn to appreciate that no one is perfect, including ourselves. We all have both positive and negative things about us. The best thing to do is to focus primarily on the positive and not the negative. Also, watch your associations. Unfortunately, sometimes we may have to break off certain questionable friendships and associations—from being around discouraging and destructive people who are overly negative and critical of us — people who knowingly or unknowingly influence us to dislike or hate ourselves. Another thing is, don't take life too seriously, learn to relax and laugh. For laughter is good medicine for the soul. And, lastly, and most importantly, view yourself as a beautiful and good person. Because that is what you are!

Weeding out bad and negative influences. Cultivating a positive attitude and spirit within us can be a lot like gardening. I'm not claiming to be a skilled plantsman or garden expert, but when it comes to gardening, common knowledge is that along with planting, watering, and fertilizing, also comes regular weeding. This is necessary because weeds can rob the soil and plants of healthy nutrients and water. And they can also choke out and destroy a healthy flower garden or crop of vegetables; depending on what it is that we are growing.

When it comes to our mind, the same can be true. Weeds (in this case, negative influences) can be harmful to our thinking, attitude, outlook, and overall health. These weeds can come in many forms. They can be influences that we let into our homes through TV programs, movies, video games, computer websites, and even certain people that we choose to associate with. So if we desire to have positive thinking and a healthy outlook, there may be certain things that we might need to be more selective about, or that we decide to completely remove from our lives that have a negative and damaging influence on us.

Roll with life's punches. As we all well know, life is not all fun and games. As a matter of fact, sometimes it can throw us some pretty hard blows so-to-speak. And, how we personally react when this happens, can make a big difference on how we fair when under fire or trial. For example, if we overreact to a situation it can make matters much worse. But when we handle matters calmly and rationally, we can often diffuse or lesson the magnitude or impact of a situation that could so easily spiral out of control. How might this be done?

Well, when dealing with life's problems sometimes it is best to just roll with the punches. For example, our family car got hit twice, on two separate occasions, both within a matter of just a short time span. As a matter of fact, we had just gotten our vehicle repaired from being in the first accident, and then a week or two later, someone ran into it again, but this time in a store parking lot. These of course were both costly and painful experiences. Also, to add insult to injury, both incidents were hit and run accidents, where the other drivers fled the scene. This was indeed both irritating and frustrating, to say the least! However, when my wife and I thought about it, we reasoned that there's nothing that we can do about it. We can't change what happened. It's a done deal. It happened, and now we must cope and deal with it. Either we can decide to get all bent out of shape over it, allowing it to get the best of us, and knock us down. Or we can say: "Oh well," and then get it fixed, and go on with our life. Well, we found that the latter is the best and healthiest choice. This way we minimize the drama, and we don't prolong any possible mental and emotional pain.

Reaping good from bad. Not every problem or negative situation that we go through in life is necessary bad for us. Sometimes our sufferings can yield positive results. For one, they can aid in helping us to develop good or valuable qualities that we did not have or possess before, which are things that can help others. For example, our personal sufferings and negative experiences can help us to become more sympathetic, understanding, and merciful to other people's situations, problems, sufferings, and pain. Having gone through similar things ourselves, we can personally relate and understand what others are possibly going through. And therefore we can become a real source of comfort and encouragement to them in their time of suffering and need.

Another thing that can be gained through sufferings and bad

experiences is that sometimes they can help us to get know ourselves better, in that through the pain or grieving process, we begin to turn inward and reflect on things more deeply, and in the process, by means of performing a thorough examination of ourselves, we discover amazing things about ourselves — hidden things that we never knew existed, such as talents, gifts, and other abilities. Interestingly, this happened to me after my mom died from breast cancer. Surprisingly, at that most grievous of times, I discovered that I have a knack for writing poetry. I even had a book of poetry published, entitled "Poems That Touch Home."

Well, thus far in our discussion on coping with bipolar depression, I've touched on the importance of a positive social environment, and also cultivating a positive attitude and healthy outlook. Next, we will consider another important subject that can also be helpful, which is having and creating an uplifting home environment.

A Positive and Uplifting Home Environment

Out of all places that we spend time at, we generally spend the majority of our time at our home. Therefore, because of this, why not create a really warm, pleasant, refreshing, relaxing, and upbuilding home environment to live in. By doing this we can add a great amount of peace and enjoyment to our lives, which can be beneficial to our overall health and happiness. So what are some things that we might do to create a refreshing and relaxing home atmosphere?

Well, for one, we can make our home feel and be more relaxing and comfortable. And we can make it look more attractive too. We can also make it smell really good. In other words, it's a matter of constructing or setting up our home environment with things that will daily feed our five human senses the things that will be healthy for our mind, body, spirit, and soul. Good and valuable things that will stimulate and create peaceful, joyful, and positive feelings and thoughts—things that will uplift our mood and spirit—things that will make us feel more peaceful, secure, relaxed, and happy. This is especially important for those who suffer from bipolar disorder, for it can help them to better cope with their depression, which often goes hand in hand with feelings of anxiety and stress.

I'm not saying that we should go all out, spending a vast fortune to make our homes plush and extravagant. I don't know about you, but like most people, I simply couldn't possibly afford it. However, if we are creative and thrifty, we can keep our needs modest, reasonable, affordable, and in good taste.

So what are some things can we do to make our home environment more comfortable and relaxing?

Use proper lighting. One thing that can help to make our home more uplifting and relaxing is by making sure that we have proper lighting, so that it is not too bright, and yet not too dim. Proper lighting is especially important for those who suffer from bipolar disorder, because their eyes are often highly sensitive to bright lights, which can make them feel irritable and uncomfortable.

Peace and quiet. It's been said "Silence is golden." Yes, a certain amount of peace and quiet is important to humans, but especially is this essential to those who are bipolar, because their ears are often highly sensitive to noise. With this in mind, if possible, sometimes it's best to free ourselves from nerve rattling sounds and disturbing chaos, by eliminating as much unnecessary noise and disturbances that we can.

Pleasant and soothing fragrances. Another thing that we can incorporate into our home atmosphere is soothing and pleasant aroma fragrances, by unitizing aroma therapy or lighting scented candles, etc. This can help to calm one's nerves and put them in a better mood. However, for those who may be allergic to certain fragrances or smells, they may need to exercise caution when it comes to choosing the right ones, or they may wish to eliminate them entirely.

Listening to relaxing music. It has been said that "Music soothes the savage beast." True, music can have a calming and peaceful affect on many things, including humans. With this in mind, occasionally, we may want to have some refreshing music playing softly in the background, to create a relaxing atmosphere and to help generate a pleasant mood.

Caution: When it comes to one's choice of music, it of course is a personal decision as to what kind we may personally choose to listen to. However, sometimes, we may need to exercise caution when it comes to selecting certain music or songs, because, depending on what it is, some can leave us feeling melancholy and blue, which can end up creating or feeding depression.

Choosing comfortable furniture. Another thing that can help our home environment to be more relaxing is by having comfortable furniture to sit on. With this in mind, you may decide to have a favorite, comfortable chair, lounge, or rocker available to sit on. Also, along with this, you may choose to have a soft, warm, and cozy throw blanket near at hand; one that you can wrap up in on cool and crisp days and nights—anything that will help you to feel relaxed, and that can aid in reducing stress.

A fireplace. A fireplace in not something that is a necessity of life, but, personally, I thought that it would be nice to have one. Unfortunately, we didn't have one built into our house. So I decided to purchase an electric one. Surprisingly, it was relatively inexpensive, and also economically affordable to run. And, believe me, it was one of the best purchases that I've ever made. I absolutely love it! There's just something about it that puts me in a relaxed and cozy mood, especially on a cold and frigid, wintery day or night in good ole Minnesnowta! So, by all means, if you don't already have a built-in fireplace, I would encourage you to take advantage of the comfort and relaxation that having an electric one can offer and provide.

Choosing uplifting décor. It is truly amazing what a little home décor can bring to a lifeless room. It can transform a dull and boring setting into a fun, uplifting, stimulating, and exciting place. With this in mind, you may decide to add some joyful and stimulating décor to your home environment, such as: beautiful and interesting artwork, portraits or pictures of people or places or things, fun and pleasant knickknacks, and other uplifting things— anything that will inspire you and make you smile and feel good. In addition to this, you may want to paint your rooms soothing colors—hues that will have a calming effect on your mood and spirit—tints that will help to relax your mind, heart, and soul.

Use of indoor plants. Indoor plants can bring natural beauty, life, and radiance to any room. Because of this, you may personally choose to incorporate some into your indoor environment. Interestingly, plants not only give off valuable oxygen, but they can also be soothing, comforting, and therapeutic too. Besides this, there is just something good about nurturing, caring for, and helping other things to be vibrant and healthy. In the process, it can have a reciprocal, good affect on us as well. It's like having a healthy interchange of encouragement and building one another up.

Maintaining a clean and clutter free environment. An un-kept and dirty living environment, along with bad odors, can add discomfort and stress to one's life. It can even feed depression. Having this in mind, we may want to try to keep our home environment as clean and clutter free as possible. For this can add not only peace, enjoyment, and comfort to our lives, but it is also good for our overall health and wellness too.

No doubt, all of the things listed above, will feed our senses (sight, smell, hearing, and touch), positive and uplifting things that will be good for our overall health and wellbeing, including our emotional and mental health. However, these are just a few suggestions. The truth is, the sky is the limit as to what you might decide to personally incorporate into your own personal home environment that will suit and satisfy your taste and needs. The important thing is that you try to make your home a miniature, refreshing oasis; one that you can escape to, especially in times of need — an environment that will produce a beautiful, peaceful, relaxing, and positive atmosphere that will uplift your spirits, and make you think and feel better.

A Healthy Diet and Life Style

In many ways, having and maintaining a healthy life style is conducive to good health. It can make a big difference in how we feel and function on a daily basis. On the other hand, when we neglect our health it can lead to various problems where we eventually feel and experience the negative effects. True, having and maintaining a healthy life style is no sure solution or guarantee that we won't ever get sick. However, when we do everything possible within our power and ability to be and stay healthy, we can to a certain degree, lessen the chance.

Our bodies are a lot like a house, in that it must be regularly and properly kept up and maintained. Because if we neglect giving it the necessary attention and preventive maintenance that it regularly requires, it will eventually get rundown and fall apart. Having this in mind, what are some things that we might do or incorporate in our life that can promote good health within us? Well, one thing is by having a good diet.

A good and healthy diet. Having and maintaining a good and healthy diet is very important for everyone. Why? Because it is good for our overall health and wellbeing. Subsequently, if we eat good and nutritious foods, we will be properly nourishing our body—providing it with the right building blocks that it needs to refuel, energize, and restore itself. On the other hand, if we were to eat and subsist primarily on unhealthy junk food, we would be starving our bodies of the healthy nutrients that it needs to function properly. But, not only that, these bad things can be detrimental to our physical health. For example, we could become obese, which can lead to developing heart disease, high blood pressure, and a host of other serious health issues.

You might ask: What is a healthy diet? Well, a good, healthy, and well-balanced diet consists of regularly eating whole grains, fruits, vegetables, protein, diary, and also good fats and sugars in proper proportions on a daily basis. If you personally happen to need help in this area, you may wish to consult your doctor or a local nutritionist, who will be more than happy to help.

Along with having and maintaining a healthy diet, we also need to make sure that we are taking in an adequate amount of something else, which is *water*.

Drink plenty of H²O. Water is truly an amazing, life sustaining substance. Interestingly, it covers about 70% of the earth's surface. And it also makes up about 70% of the human body. The fact is, water is an essential and vital element to all life forms. It not only keeps us alive, but it's refreshing, it tastes good, and it is healthy for us too. For example, it helps our bodily organs to function properly. And it aids in proper blood circulation and digestion. It also helps to flush harmful toxins from our bodies. Another amazing thing is that water has zero calories. Because of this it can also aid in weight control and weight loss.

With all of the good benefits that water supplies, it is wise to make sure that we keep properly hydrated. Personally, I drink about a gallon of water daily.[60]

Note: If you exercise, you will need to factor this in to your water intake needs, so that you will be and stay properly hydrated. Because exercise will naturally deplete water from your body through sweating. To help you to properly monitor your water intake levels, you might choose to use a water intake calculator to help you to calculate your personal daily needs. Interestingly, some water intake calculators are available online for free. All you need to do is find one on an appropriate website; plug in your weight; and your total daily workout time, and it will automatically calculate your targeted daily water intake for you. It's that simple!

Another thing that can aid in having good health is by riding our bodies of harmful toxins.

----

[60] Caution: Because some people have medical conditions such as heart, and kidney issues, etc... that may limit their water intake needs, be sure to check with your doctor, and then follow his or her recommendations.

Rid your mind and body of harmful toxins. Another thing that is good for one's health and that can help us feel better, is to periodically detox our body of unhealthy toxins and other harmful substances. There are many ways that this can be done. One way is by periodically doing a weekend cleanse by eating natural detoxifying foods. Another way is by preparing certain green drinks that have a detoxifying effect.

Another way to detox is by using a Sauna. Any sauna will be useful and helpful. However, I've personally found that infrared saunas are one of the best, because the infrared heat absorbs or penetrates deeper into human tissue, producing more sweat than other saunas, which is a highly efficient and effective way of removing unwanted toxins from the body. Another good thing about infrared saunas is that, not only are they safe, but they are also very refreshing and relaxing.

Another way to help rid our bodies of unhealthy toxins is by drinking plenty of freshwater. Because water is a natural way of helping our bodies to cleanse themselves and flush impurities and toxins out of our system.

Another effective thing that can help to detox our bodies is by eliminating unhealthy foods from our diet. Personally, one thing in particular that has helped me was by totally eliminating refined sugar from my diet. The truth is refined sugar is not good for any of us.

Totally eliminating refined sugar from one's diet may seem a bit excessive to some people. And, of course, it is something that you don't have to personally do. However, the main reason why I decided to do it, is because I was consuming too much of it. Also, I just couldn't seem to gain control over it. So for my own personal sake and immediate health I decided that it was best for me to eliminate it entirely.

Prior to eliminating sugar from my diet, I had a huge sweet tooth. I pretty much loved any and everything that had sugar in it. I was a sugarholic, a true sugar junkie! There was a point when I was drinking anywhere from upwards to 6 to 8 cans of soda pop daily. And that was just soda, not to mention the cookies, donuts, cakes, ice cream, candy, and other items that contained sugar that I was also frequently consuming. The bad thing is, not only was this bad for my overall health, but it also put me in danger of being a borderline diabetic. In addition to this, it also caused me to put on a lot of weight. However, the good thing is that when I discontinued eating sugar, and started eating right, by implementing a good and healthy diet into my life, along with exercise; my health quickly improved. Interestingly, within the first four months of my diet, I lost 32 pounds! And I have continued to lose weight ever since. Another good benefit is that it made me very happy the day when I was able to fit back into my clothes and dress suites that I had grown out of in the past.

Another good and important thing that cutting sugar from my diet did, was that it helped my moods to become more stable, for I no longer have the sugar highs and lows. But the most important thing that I have gained is that I am no longer a borderline diabetic!

True, eliminating sugar from one's diet is not an easy thing to do. It takes a lot of sacrifice and willpower. One reason why is because there is sugar in practically everything! Another reason why is because there are also many temptations to deal with — like when we are out shopping at the local grocery stores. Interestingly, grocery stores are advertising experts; they know exactly what items are the big sellers, and what things will attract our attention. So they conveniently place and locate these items where they are sure to catch our eye. Often, the moment we enter the grocery store, the first thing that we are greeted with at the entryway door is sugar products, such as: soda pop, freshly baked bakery items, chips, candies, etc... so that we will see and be tempted to buy them. The reason why is because stores make a lot of money on these things. Unfortunately, because of this, a person that is on a special diet has to have strong willpower to say no to these things, which is not always an easy thing to do.

After I first started my sugar free diet, I vividly recall that after being without sugar for five days, I suffered withdrawal symptoms, which left me feeling extremely irritable, crabby, and anxious. However, by the eighth day these symptoms went away for good. One thing that helped was that I replaced refined sugar with natural fruits, such as grapes, pineapple, oranges, watermelons, bananas, apples, plums, etc. Interestingly, now, after being off of sugar for so long, I find that fruits taste even better than they did in the past!

Another thing that helped me in my resolve to stay off sugar, was that before I went on my sugar free diet, I condition my mind in advance (for a considerable length of time) to stick to my decision, so that once I started my diet, I would be determined to stay off of sugar. This way, if pastries and other sugar products are waved under my nose or they are in the house for other family members to eat, they won't tempt me to eat or consume them.

Sugar is just one thing that one may choose to eliminate or reduce the amount of from their diet. There are many other foods and things that one can choose to either permanently or periodically eliminate from their diet that can help them to successfully detox their body.

In addition to detoxifying our bodies of harmful toxins, another important thing that we can do to encourage and promote good health in us, is by incorporating *exercise* into our lives.

Exercise regularly. When it comes to exercise, it is not only good for our physical health, but it is also very important to our emotional and mental health too. So if you haven't already done so, why not try starting and maintaining a regular weekly exercise program. The truth is there are many health benefits associated with exercise. Some of them are: (1) It increases circulation of oxygen and blood flow to the body and brain, (2) It is an excellent stress reducer, (3) It helps rid our bodies of harmful chemicals and toxins, (4) It can boost our immune system, (5) It releases natural chemicals such as endorphins, dopamine, norepinephrine, and serotonin in the brain—things that will help us to be and feel better, (6) It can help us to sleep better at night, (7) It can aid in helping us to shed unwanted pounds, and, lastly, (8) It can help us to feel more positive, confident, and better about ourselves.[61]

Get plenty of sleep. Another thing that is good for one's health and wellbeing is to get an adequate amount of sleep — preferably eight hours per night. Because sleep helps our bodies to recover and be energized and recharged for the next day. Without the adequate amount of sleep our mind and bodies cannot function properly. Nor will we have the energy, focus, and stamina that we need to perform at our highest levels.

Purchase a good bed, and shoes. On average, we as humans spend about 8 hours per night sleeping, which basically amounts to about one third of our lives. Because of this, it is important to have a good and comfortable bed, so that we can get a good night's sleep. True, a good bed can be a very costly purchase. However, it's been said that there are two things in life that a person should never skimp on when it comes to cost or price, and that is: (1) a good and comfortable bed and, (2) a good, supportive pair of shoes. The reason why is because we spend the majority of our time in them. For when you think about it, if we are not in the one, we are in the other.

As respects beds, the reason why it is so vitally important to have a good, quality one, is that it can make a world of difference, as far as the *quality* of sleep that we get each night. Some good benefits of this is that it can truly refresh us, making us feel less stressful, more alert, energetic, alive, and ready to tackle another eventful and challenging day.

In regards to our feet, we can say that to a certain degree and in many ways that they are the pathways to good health. For example, if we weren't to take good care of our feet, it could cause us to develop various health issues, such as a leg, or back problems, etc, which can wind up being very disruptive to our sleep, and also cripple our ability to be able to function and perform certain daily tasks and engage in many fun and enjoyable activities. Therefore,

---

[61] Before starting an exercise program it is always best to consult with your doctor first.

having this in mind, doesn't it make sense to protect and take good care of our feet the best way that we can, in particular, by wearing proper and comfortable shoes.

Having highlighted the good benefits of the two valuable things mentioned above (bed and shoes), we can see why it is important to purchase and have both a good bed and shoes.

Take advantage of sunshine. The sun, which is located some 93 million miles away from planet earth, exerts a powerful influence on our lives. As a direct result, many people throughout history have become devoted sun worshipers. Today, there are the dedicated sunbathers who regularly seek to acquire that all so appealing and fashionable Coppertone tan. Also, there's the annual vacationers in North America who yearly migrate south during the cold winter months, to the highly attractive sunshine state of Florida, U.S.A, in order to enjoy the warm weather and bask in the rays of the beautiful sun.[62] Truly, from all of this, we can undeniably see that the sun is very attractive and highly important to us as humans.

You might ask: Why are people so fascinated and attracted to the sun? Well, the reason why is because in many ways it is good for our health. In what ways? Well, a couple important and valuable things that the sun does for us, is that it lifts us up emotionally, and it energizes us. Another thing is that it provides valuable Vitamin D, something that our bodies require and that aids in keeping us feeling good and happy. Interestingly, there are many people who suffer from Seasonal Affective Disorder (SAD). This is due to experiencing a lack of sunshine during fall and winter seasons, when there are not as many sunny days, due to cloudy, overcast skies. Subsequently, as a result of this, we can definitely see that the sun can exert a healthy and powerful

---

[62] Caution: Although the sun can have a positive and good affect on our emotions and so forth, on the flipside of things it can also be harmful (causing skin cancer) if we don't take necessary precautions, such as wearing proper clothing, applying proper sunscreen lotion, etc. when being exposed to its ultraviolet rays.

influence on our lives, especially on our moods and mental health.

What might one personally do to combat SAD during gloomy, cloudy, overcast seasons? One thing that might help is by taking a Vitamin D supplement to compensate for a lack of sunshine. Another thing that often helps is by using light therapy or a SAD lamp. Light therapy uses artificial light that mimics natural sunlight. This can be an effective way to treat SAD and certain other conditions. True, light therapy lamps can be expensive. The good thing is they are often paid for by one's medical insurance company. However, if medical insurance won't approve or pay for it, or you don't happen to have insurance — depending on where you shop, it can be purchased for a somewhat reasonable price online. So, if by chance you happen to want or you are in need of purchasing a SAD lamp, make sure that you do your research and shop around for both a good price and a good quality lamp (one that delivers the recommended 10,000 LUX light therapy), before you decide to purchase or buy.[63]

From all of this, we can see that whenever possible, that it is important to take full advantage of the healthy and curative aspects of the sun and the natural light that it provides, especially if we happen to suffer from depression. In regards to sunlight, to both our enjoyment and delight, my wife and I recently moved into a home that is surrounded by large windows. And, because the house conveniently faces towards the east, it brings in a lot of natural light, which makes the inside of our home always bright and cheery, especially on sunny days. And believe me, it makes a world of difference in regards to affecting and influencing one's mood in a positive and uplifting way.

Personal cleanliness and proper grooming. It has been said that "Cleanliness is next to godliness." This includes not only the

---

[63] Caution: Before taking Vitamin D supplements, or using a light therapy, SAD lamp, be sure to check with your doctor beforehand to make sure that these things are right for you personally. Also, he or she may want to monitor the dosage of Vitamin D, or the time and frequency of the use of a Light Therapy Lamp.

physical cleanliness of our homes, and cars, etc., but also the personal cleanliness of our bodies. Yes, good personal hygiene and proper grooming are very important. They can have, not only a positive effect on how we feel about ourselves, but they can also give us a certain amount of dignity and self respect. But more importantly it is also good for our health and wellbeing. Just think about what could happen if we were to never brush our teeth. Eventually they would rot and fall out. Also, if we were never to bathe and wash ourselves, it can lead to having body sores and infectious diseases. And just think of the bad odors all of this would produce. In the process we would lose a lot of friends, because nobody would want to be around us. How much better we and others are when we give appropriate attention to personal cleanliness and good grooming.

Learn to relax. Life can be stressful. Not only is this true, but it's probably a gross understatement. For many have to daily cope with things such as earning a living, rush hour traffic, pressures in school or on the job, the everyday hustle and bustle of life, and so forth. Because of these things, tensions and stress levels can so easily build and flare up in us, which, if we are not careful, can lead to serious health issues. Knowing this, it is absolutely vital for us to seek and find things that can help us to relax and unwind. What kind of things might help? Well, there are a vast number of things that we can choose from that can help us to de-stress. Things such as getting away and taking a needed vacation, or getting a body massage, or using a steam room or a sauna, or sitting in a whirlpool, or utilizing aromatherapy, or taking a peaceful and quiet stroll through nature's woodlands or a local park, or reading a good book, or gardening, or going fishing, etc— anything that we can utilize that will help us to unwind and relax.

Take Time to Breathe. From the very moment of birth — when we took our first breath of fresh air — it has been essential for us to breathe. This is both a necessary and vital function of life. For not only does it keep us alive, but it also serves other purposes as well, such as providing us with the oxygen that our bodies require to properly manage and regulate itself, so as to keep us healthy. For example, the oxygen that we take in flushes toxins, such as carbon dioxide out of our body. It also burns sugars and fatty acids in our cells to produce energy. These are just a couple of the valuable things that breathing does for us, there are more.

In addition to helping our physical bodies to stay healthy, breathing can also play an important role in our emotional health too, especially if we both learn how to and practice breathing right, which involves deep diaphragmatic breathing.[64] One of benefits of doing this is that it can help to relieve stress and anxiety, which in turn, can make us feel better mentally, emotionally, as well as physically.

Because breathing is so vitally important to our overall health and well-being, it would be advantageous for us to set aside some personal time (preferably 10 to 20 minute per day), to engage in breathing exercises. By doing this, we will feel so much better.

Take one day at a time. Often, it can be difficult for people with bipolar disorder to be able to function normally on a daily basis, by performing simple daily tasks. In this regards, sometimes it is best not to get too worked up over worrying about what tomorrow or the future will bring. But, instead, learn to relax, by taking just one day at a time. This can help one to avoid feeling too overwhelmed! The truth is, life has enough pressures and problems for us to deal with as it is, coupled with daily anxieties. A person doesn't need to add to this by putting too much of a load on themselves. So just learn to relax, by taking one day at a time, by doing this it can take a huge weight off of one's shoulders.

Help and Support from Family and Friends

As humans, we all need a good, positive, and loving support base (people that we can approach, or those that we have around who can encourage us, uplift our spirit, and make us feel good about ourselves and life). This is absolutely essential, especially

---

[64] For those of us that need help with breathing exercises and the techniques on how to breathe correctly, you can either consult a physician, or check out several good and helpful instructional videos online.

when we happen to be undergoing difficult and troubling times. This is where friends and family support in particular can come in real handy.

Personally, I can attest to how encouraging others have been to me, especially my wife, children, and family members. For example, when I was hospitalized in the past for having severe depression, they were not only there for me, but they were also very loving and supportive. Quickly rallying together, they came to my immediate aid, showing kindness, understanding, patience, and rendering helpful and positive assistance. And even though I was completely overwhelmed with sadness at the time, it made me feel good and secure having them in my corner and by my side.

Interestingly, encouraging words, whether they are written or spoken, can be extremely powerful and helpful. They can have a soothing, healing, and cheering affect upon one's mind, heart, and soul, thereby lifting and picking them up during difficult, discouraging, and hard times. On the other hand, negative speech, along with a lack of support and encouragement can cause and feed sadness, and even deep depression.

Often, when it comes to dealing with the distressing pain of bipolar disorder, there are times when one has the tendency to isolate themselves from others. Sometimes, this can go on for days, and weeks. Unfortunately, this happened to me shortly after I had suffered a mental breakdown. Finally, my wife had to intervene and encourage me to seek immediate medical help, which I did. Fortunately for me, if it wasn't for her loving help, encouragement, and support, who knows how bad things might have gotten. Whatever the case, this shows how important it is for us not to completely isolate ourselves from others, especially from those who can encourage and support us during times of need.

Setting Positive Goals

Having both short term and long term goals is important. The reason why is because they help to keep us motivated and moving forward in life. Without goals, are lives can easily become stagnated and unfulfilled. Yes, goals are important for everybody, but especially are they good and healthy for people who suffer from depression. Speaking from personal experience, it is so easy to become so weighed down and engulfed in one's emotional pain and sorrows that in the process we let life slip away or pass us by.

So if you personally don't have any goals that you are currently working on, why not start one today. It doesn't have to be anything huge or complicated. It could be the simple goal of exercising for 10 minutes, three times a week. And then, after you get use to this, perhaps later, you might want to gradually increase the amount of your workout time, until you get to 30 minutes workouts, three times per week.

Sometimes, it is best to keep our goals simple, realistic, and obtainable, rather than setting the bar too high so to speak, only to fall short of reaching them, which in itself can be highly discouraging.

So don't sit idle and let life pass you by. But, instead, be determined to make the most of it, by having and setting reachable and attainable goals that keep you, not only moving forward, but also feeling proud and good about yourself, your personal achievements, and accomplishments.

Being Conscious of Your Spiritual Needs

As humans, we were created with a need, not only for physical food and things, but equally important, if not even more so, is the fact that we also have a spiritual need too. And by reaching out to fulfill and satisfy that need, it helps to contribute, not only to good spiritual health, but also to good emotional, mental, and physical health too. The reason being is because all of these things happen to be interdependently linked together. With that being said, what are some things that being spiritual can do for us?

Happiness. One important thing that being spiritual does for a person, is that it contributes to their happiness. Interestingly, during his famous Sermon on the Mount speech, God's son, Jesus Christ, said: "Happy are those conscious of their spiritual need!" (Matthew 5:3) Yes, by both recognizing the need for and seeking God's guidance, it contributes to real contentment, a sense of satisfaction, and fulfillment in life, which can individually bring us a good measure of personal happiness.

Comfort during times of need. Another thing that being spiritual can do for us, is that we can gain peace and comfort through prayer, especially during times of need. At 2 Corinthians 1:3, 4 it says: "3 Praised be the God and Father of our Lord Jesus Christ, the Father of tender mercies and the God of all comfort, 4 who comforts us in all our trials so that we may be able to comfort others in any sort of trial with the comfort that we receive from God."

Valuable fruits of the God's spirit. Some additional benefits that we can gain through spirituality, is that the Holy Spirit, which we receive from God, can produce joy and other valuable qualities in us, qualities that can help us to endure trials and sufferings. At Galatians 5:22, 23 it says: "22 On the other hand, the fruitage of the spirit is love, joy, peace, patience, kindness, goodness, faith, 23 mildness, and self-control."

Refreshment for our souls. God's son, Jesus Christ, invitingly encourages us at Matthew 11:28, 29, saying: "28 Come to me, all you who are toiling and loaded down, and I will refresh you. 29 Take my yoke upon you and learn from me, for I am mild-tempered and lowly in heart, and you will find refreshment for yourselves. 30 For my yoke is kindly, and my load is light."

Relief from burdens. Life is an amazing, wonderful, and beautiful thing. But it also has its share of troubles and problems too. However, lucky for us, we are not alone in having to deal with them. For God willingly and generously offers to help carry our heavy burdens for us. At Psalm 55:22, we are encouraged: "Throw your burden on Jehovah, and he will sustain you. Never will he allow the righteous one to fall."

Positive hope for the future. In regards to those who may currently be suffering from a discouraging illness, the Bible gives positive encouragement and hope. Concerning a future time, so near at hand, God promises to cure all sicknesses and diseases, Isaiah 33:24 says about that coming time period: "24 And no resident will say: I am sick. The people dwelling in the land will be pardoned for their error." What a truly amazing time this will be, when people are no longer sick!

Yes, as we can see from the above examples, there are many helpful and wonderful things that we can gain from being conscious of our spiritual need.

In conclusion, from all of the things that we just considered in this chapter of my book, we can clearly see that there are many things that one can personally take advantage of and do that can aid in helping them to successfully cope with bipolar disorder. For a condensed list of some of these, as well as additional, helpful things, please see the information "A Recipe for a Healthy Mind," on pages 196-197. And also, "Things That Can Help Fight Added Depression," on pages 198-201.

A Recipe for a Healthy Mind

1. View yourself as a beautiful and good person.

2. Stay positive, by feeding your mind positive and up-building things.

3. Don't completely isolate yourself from others.

4. Associate with optimistic, encouraging, helpful, and happy people.

5. Be forgiving.

6. Always look for the good in people and things, even when it doesn't seem to be there.

7. Get plenty of rest and sleep.

8. Have and maintain a good and healthy nutritious diet.

9. Drink plenty of water. Because water promotes good health and helps to flush harmful toxins out of our system.

10. Avoid consuming too much refined sugar. This can be bad for one's overall health.

11. Exercise regularly. It's important to have a consistent, weekly exercise program in place. Caution: Be sure to check with your Doctor first before starting an exercise program, and then follow his or her suggestions and recommendations.

12. Get plenty of sunshine. Or during cloudy seasons, such as wintertime, when the sun doesn't come out as much, you may want to take a Vitamin D supplement. Or, if possible, use Light Therapy (a SAD lamp). Caution: Be sure to use appropriate sunscreen when exposed to the sun. Also, when it comes to Vitamin D supplements or Light Therapy, be sure to consult your doctor to determine what is best for you.

13. Have and set good and healthy obtainable goals.

14. Set limitations. It's important to know your limitations, and to set boundaries. This way you won't be spreading yourself too thin or be biting off more than you can personally handle or

chew, which can result in inflicting unnecessary stress and anxiety on ourselves.

15. Practice giving. The Bible says: "There is more happiness in giving than there is in receiving." (Acts 20:35)

16. Make time for recreation and play.

17. Don't vegetate mainly on TV or surfing the internet. Instead, you might want to find a good book to read. Or do some other fun and creative things.

18. Release daily stress. You can do this by using and having stress reducers in place. There are many options to choose from. Find what works best for you.

19. Learn to relax and breathe.

20. Take one day at a time.

The things listed above may seem like a lot to do and apply at first. But don't worry. Don't let this overwhelm you. Instead, you might want to incorporate just one thing at a time into your daily routine. And then, when you become comfortable with it, you might want to slowly and progressively add more. Keep in mind that even if you do just a little, it is more beneficial than not doing anything at all.[65]

---

[65] This is not to say that if a person applies these things that they as a result will have a perfectly healthy mind. However, it can to a certain degree be beneficial and helpful when we personally do all that we can to lead good and healthy lives.

Things That Can Help Fight Added Depression

Do's & Don'ts: Listed below in no specific order:

- Don't become a product of negative thought. But, instead, fight it! This is important because often our thinking has the power to dictate who we are or what we become.

- Do not expect or look to receive approval from everyone. It may never happen!

- Don't blame yourself for having bipolar disorder. It is not your fault. It's a disease, like cancer or any other illness. Nor is it due to your being mentally or spiritually weak as some ignorant or highly uninformed people might imply. It is just a malady or illness that people happened to get. So don't punish yourself. Also, you are not a bad person because you suffer from depression or bipolar disorder. It can happen to anybody.

- Don't expect or wait for anybody to help you with your mental health condition. The balls in your court. So take the initiative to seek and get the medical help and any other assistance that you may need.

- Don't stop taking your prescribed medications, unless it is recommended by your doctor. Otherwise this can cause a mental relapse.

- Do not place yourself in an overly negative and critical environment that aggravates and feeds your depression.

- Do not completely isolate yourself from others. As humans, we were created or made to be social creatures that both need and can positively feed off of others.

- Don't hold grudges by keeping account of the injury or pain that others may have inflicted upon you. It is better to forgive, even if the wrongs that people commit against us seem intentional. Why? Because resentment and hate can be harmful and damaging to our emotional, mental, and physical health.

- "Do not let yourself be conquered by the evil, but keep conquering the evil with the good." (Romans 12:21)

- Don't be overly negative and critical of others. The fact is we can find faults and weaknesses in everyone, including ourselves. We all have them. The reason being is that we are all sinful, imperfect creatures. The challenging thing is to look for and focus on the good in people and things. If we practice doing this it will be good for us and others, including our own health.

- Don't let depression control you. Take control of the steering wheel so-to-speak, and guide and steer yourself in a positive and uplifting direction.

- Don't expect perfection or too much from others. Also, don't put anyone on too high of a pedestal. Have reasonable expectations and opinions of people. This way you won't be too devastated or let down if they should happen to disappoint you.

- Don't let your shortcomings discourage and crush you. But rather, view your mistakes and negative experiences as valuable stepping stones of positive learning experiences that: *(1) Will help to improve your outlook on life, and (2) Will aid in improving and strengthening your value and character, and (3) Will help to prepare you for a better future* — rather than viewing them as stumbling blocks of hurt and pain, which can cripple your growth, development, forward momentum, and progress, as well as rob you of inner peace, joy, and happiness.

- Don't let others decide and dictate your personal value or self-worth. Instead, accept and appreciate yourself for the beautiful and valuable person that you are.

- Don't beat yourself up over past mistakes. True, it is normal to feel bad about the shortcomings and errors that we have made in life, especially big ones. But too much guilt can crush one's spirit. It can also rob us of our inner peace, joy, and happiness. The truth is, we cannot correct or change our past. But we can learn from our mistakes and move forward. You will feel so much better for doing this.

- Don't let others keep punishing you for your past mistakes. I call this type of fault-finding, which is often accompanied by nasty verbal assaults, the "You did this, and you did that syndrome." This type of fault-finding or finger pointing is when someone never lets you forget the past. But rather, they keep bringing it up, over and over again, constantly throwing it in your face; causing you to re-live the pain over and over again. The fact is, for the overall health and benefit of both us and them, they need to get over it, and so do we. For finger pointing can be highly crippling and damaging to both the recipient and their friendship or relationship with others. But it can also make life truly miserable!

- Do not allow your mind free reign to think as it wants. But instead, exercise self control and discipline. Like driving a moving vehicle, we must take and maintain control of the wheel by guiding and steering our minds in a positive direction to where we want it to go.

- Don't let bad feelings or emotions get the best of you. The fact is bad feelings and emotions can drown or bury us if we allow them to. But also, they can make us sick (emotionally, mentally, and physically). So don't let them overwhelm you. Instead, take and keep control over them.

- Don't over-think things. Sometimes, if we dig too deep, especially in regards to negative things, it can create unnecessary problems, which can lead us into a sinkhole of misery and despair.

- Don't let the hypocrisy of others discourage you.

- Don't keep or pursue hurtful, discouraging, or worthless, so called "friends." They will only pull you down. So cut them off and let them go. And then move onto seeking positive associates that will love, encourage, support, and build you up.

- Don't sit idle for too long. Try to stay busy. For it's been said "An idle mind is the devil's playground." Also, inactivity can be harmful to us to a certain degree, in that it can zap us of our energy, causing us to become more sluggish, and even depressed. On the other hand, being active in good pursuits can energize us—giving us even more energy! Also, it can aid in helping us to have a more positive viewpoint and outlook about ourselves! So try to stay busy if you can.

- Don't feel sorry for yourself. Too much self pity can be self-destructive and damaging.

- Don't let the overly negative and critical opinions and viewpoints of others discourage and tear you down. The truth is there are much better and more uplifting things in life to concentrate and focus your valuable time, energy, and attention on.

- Don't let others emotionally abuse you. Unfortunately, there are some sick people in the world who get their kicks out of verbally crushing and abusing others. However, for your own emotional and mental health, and overall well-being, get away from them ASAP, and avoid them like the plague!

- Don't let others judge or determine your personal standing with God. The truth is, sometimes people can be overly negative and critical, self-righteous, and condemning. But, ultimately, the decision lies with God. It is up to him to judge and decide your fate and standing with him.

- Do not self-medicate. Unfortunately, some people try to drown their sorrows and pain in alcohol, or illicit drug use, etc. But in the end these crippling and self damaging pursuits wind up leaving them feeling empty and even more depressed.

- Don't give up. As difficult as life can sometimes seem, it is still worth living. And often circumstances or things that at present may seem completely lost and hopeless, oftentimes they can and do change for the better. So keep hope alive. For hope is like a bright beacon that brightens our path and enlightens our way!

Chapter 8

LESSONS LEARNED

AND

THE ROAD AHEAD

Along the long, and often challenging road of life, there are many twists and turns. Because of this, we really don't know for a certainty what truly lies ahead of us, or what tomorrow will bring. Along with the good, sometimes there will also be bad. But, overall, life is a delightfully curious and beautiful thing. And we should cherish and take advantage of every moment that we can. True, we will have a certain measure of problems; some might even be serious health issues. However, if we can find and use positive and effective ways to deal with them, it can make a world of difference in helping us to successfully cope.

Personally, I have learned many things in life, mostly through experience. And I have a lot more to learn. Nevertheless, this is all good, because hopefully I can use the valuable lessons that I've gained, not only to benefit myself, but also to encourage and help others who are undergoing similar experiences and problems, like bipolar disorder.

What are some of the things that I've learned?

Lessons Learned

In looking back at the past, I've learned in regards to my individual situation or case, that "environment" is the primary cause of my bipolar disorder (a theory that I initially set out to prove at the beginning of this book).[66] Notably, this illness developed over an extended period of time; through a series of stages, which were: (1) *bouts of depression,* (2) that gradually and progressively escalated to *chronic depression or mental illness,* (3) which, in turn, led to an *emotional trauma* that finally triggered *bipolar disorder.*[67]

I have also learned that a large portion of the emotional stress and depression that I have experienced in life was initiated, fueled, and fed by the "false image" of the African American that was created during the time of institutional black slavery in America — a damaging and hurtful, negative image, which I (and other descendants of slaves) have inherited, and been forced to carry throughout my entire life. And also by the oppressive, discriminatory, and ostracized treatment that I've often had to cope and deal with at the hands of both the white and black races.

---

[66] "Environment," meaning: All of the external factors that have a formative influence on a person's physical, mental, emotional, and moral development. Note: I believe that "Environment" is the main ingredient or factor that contributed to me having and developing bipolar disorder, which my life clearly proves.

[67] An important thing to note is that whatever it may be that creates or causes mental illness or bipolar disorder in one person (although others may be exposed to the same conditions or situations); it may not necessarily cause it in someone else. The reason being is because we are all separate individuals with different internal makeup's and characteristics. And what affects one person a certain way, may affect someone else completely different, or perhaps, not at all.

To be truthful, this has been a very hard and difficult journey for me. For being a victim of injustice was a stumbling block to me in certain ways, just as it is to so many others. It brought me a lot of heartache, pain and suffering. Also, to a certain extent it crippled my potential development and forward momentum and advancement in certain ways. I'm not using this as an excuse or anything for things that I may have failed to realize or achieve, for I feel that I have lived a fairly successful and fulfilling life to a large degree. It's just that, as of lately, I'm now trying to piece together what caused my illness, so that I can pull things together, to start the healing and recovery process, in order to get on with my life and to make the most of what is left. The truth is, many times the root cause of a person's problem or situation is the very thing that is zapping their power and strength. Sometimes, you have to find what the root source of the problem is, before you can clearly see the solution that will release you from the burden of disorientation and pain — in order to put you on the right path.

Luckily, for me, now that I know the root cause of my bipolar disorder, knowledge of this brings me a certain measure of comfort and relief. And it helps me to better cope with my illness. Also, this acquired knowledge has helped me to formulate a strategy and plan — to develop and put together the effective tools, which I detailed and highlighted in chapter seven of this book, that I need to utilize to help me cope with my situation and depression, so that I can possibly slowdown or stop any further emotional pain and suffering that might have resulted if these helpful things were not put into place. In other words, I finally have stopped the bleeding. And now I can work on the recovery and healing process.

Unfortunately, growing up, I never fully understood or realized the bad and harmful effects that racism was having on me personally. True, I recognized that there was a serious problem in this area in general, primarily against people of the black race, but I didn't know that it was having such a devastating effect on my emotional and mental health. And that left unchecked, it was only progressively getting worse with the passing of time. The good thing is now that I have gotten to the root cause of the problem, and I know why it is happening, and I have opened up and freely spoken about it, I am no longer troubled over the injustices that I have experienced in the past, or about those that I might undergo now and in the future. And neither do I feel resentment or anger. Finally, I can now totally put all of this behind me and successfully move on with my life.

I also have learned that I have to be the main contributor and advocate of my own overall health — including my mental and emotional health. And that throughout my life, I need to continue to follow my helpful plan and suggestions that I outlined in chapter seven of this book. Primarily, things such as: selectively choosing to be in a positive and uplifting social and home environment; striving to have and maintain positive thinking and a healthy outlook; having in place a good, balanced diet and regular exercise program; getting the proper amount of rest and sleep; and seeking the loving support and encouragement from family and friends. True, it's not that these things will necessarily remove my illness, but at least they can possibly help the road ahead to be a little more smoother, endurable, and manageable.

In an attempt to try to heal myself, I have also discovered from my own personal experience and through experimentation on myself; that when it comes to treating bipolar disorder that it's best and more effective to treat, not just one aspect of the illness, such as the mental health part alone, but rather, the entire human being. This includes the mental aspect of course, but also the emotional, physical, and spiritual part of the individual as well. That is the reason why I came up with and developed my extensive, detailed plan of attack in chapter seven.

Some of the other things that I have learned, which are listed below in no particular or special order are:

I've learned that being a victim of injustice can totally paralyze a person mentally, emotionally, and spiritually. Because the hurt and pain of being treated unjustly can completely consume one's thinking. This makes perfect since because in reality, the human mind is a lot like a radio, in that it can only tune into one channel or station at one time. If this is happening to you, don't let yourself be conquered by the evil, but instead, keep conquering the evil with good. Don't let society or people dictate who you are or what you will become. Don't let them kill or destroy the good that is in you. But rather, subject yourself to the qualities of peace, love, joy, kindness, and goodness. Let these things consume and overflow in your mind, heart, and soul. If you do, you will be much better off and happier for doing so.

I've learned that there are many things in life that we simply don't have control over. And that there are certain things that we don't have the ability or power to change. However, we do have the choice to decide how much or little we allow things to affect and influence us—for good or bad.

I've learned that we must never let the overly critical and negative viewpoints, mindsets, bias attitudes, and opinions of others (even though these may be ever so pervasive or prevalent throughout society, or a particular community, etc.) dictate and destroy the true character and beauty of the person that we are inside.

I've also learned and discovered within myself, something that's completely new, which is the thought that the distinct personality or traits that each person possesses, often dictates how greatly or deeply they are personally effected or influenced by a particular matter or thing (whether it be for good or bad). For example, as regards my situation or case of being bipolar, I believe that my innate traits or personality made me more sensitive to my negative environment, which made me more susceptible to depression, which ultimately led to bipolar disorder. Whereas, respects someone else, who has a completely different personality, who was also exposed to the exact, same environment that I was, they, because of their different personality, may not necessary be affected the same way or as deeply as I was, so as to become mentally ill.[68]

---

[68] This is a thought that I completely came up with on my own. I did not read about it or hear from anyone else.

I've have also learned that when it comes to dealing with injustices or a discriminatory structure of things in the world or society, that sometimes the best way of coping with it, is to just accept it for what it is, and then go on with your life, making the most of a negative or bad situation. And, in the process, if something different, positive, and better from what we imagined or expected eventually happens to come our way, then it's icing on the cake. The reason being is that we often don't have the ability or power to change certain things in life, especially those that are deeply woven or solidly fixed into the structure of a rigid, adamant and unchangeable thing.

The problem is, if we become discontented or upset with our present allotment or place in this world, to the point of allowing it to bend us completely out of shape so to speak; we can wind up becoming so angry, miserable, and self-consumed that it can cause to lose our focus on the more important things in life, such as being with and enjoying the beauty of our loved ones and family. Also, in addition to focusing our attention on our family, I've learned that it's good to find and focus our mind, energies, and talents on things that we are good at; things that not only can help ourselves, but that can also be used to help others too; rather than zeroing in on and focusing on negative and bad. In other words, living and engaging ourselves in a simple life that is free of emotional drama and stress, is by far the wisest and best choice.

I have also learned from experience that there are certain situations, areas, and things in life that can initiate, feed, and breed depression in us, and therefore, for our own overall health and wellbeing, we need to be ever cognizant and attuned to what these might be. And if it happens to be within our ability and power to control or change them, then we need to take the appropriate steps or actions to either minimize the negative and harmful effects that they have on us personally or to remove them entirely.

Another important thing that I have learned from experience is how bad and negative feeling and emotions can be highly discouraging and damaging to us personally, and that to protect and safeguard our emotional, mental, and physical health, we must gain control over them, by not allowing them free reign. One thing in particular that can help in this regards, is by being forgiving of others when they say or do things that hurt us, whether they happen to do this intentionally or unintentionally. Unfortunately, the problem with many of us is that we continue to harbor or hold on to things that hurt us in our youth or past; highly disturbing and troubling things that often leave emotional scars so to speak... things that keep resurfacing—that never seem to go away. Sometimes these things can linger on and on for too many years! Sad to say, in the end, we often wind up doing nothing but hurting ourselves.

In the past, if I had known what I know today, I would have made more of a conscience effort to forgive the errors of others, rather than dwelling and focusing upon the hurt that they caused. Interestingly, at the time, I honestly felt or thought that I had done this, but in reality I really hadn't. Instead, I unconsciously placed them somewhere deep inside of me, where they could simmer and further grow, only to resurface sometime later. And then, these things, along with additional, added future pains, amassed into one overwhelming, large problem. In the end, it became the "Snowball effect" of accumulating problems that eventually became too heavy of a weight and load for me to carry and bear, with the end result being, a stunning, devastating, and hurtful mental breakdown or collapse. So the advice I now give to others is, *learn to forgive and forget.* If you do this, it will spare you a lot of stress, heartache and pain.

The truth is, mainly focusing on what is bad or negative is not good, for it can harm or even destroy us if we allow it to. It can cause resentment, anger, sadness, and even depression, which can rob us of our inner peace, joy and happiness. The good and encouraging thing is, if this has happen to us personally, it is fixable. For there are positive and helpful things that we can do or implement into our lives that can help to change things for the better, both now and for all time. And they are:

- Freely forgive others, and then move on (this means to totally forgive).

- Change your thinking from negative to positive.

- Get and stay busy in productive, healthy, and positive activities and pursuits.

One useful thing that I have now, which I didn't possess before, is that I have come to recognize and know what the overall structural makeup of this world and society is and also its true character and mindset, in regards to how it often views and treats people like me. The advantage of this is that I can now use this gained knowledge to help me to navigate through the ruff and challenging areas of life. This way, I can perhaps ward off or soften any hurtful insults and blows or unjust treatment that may come my way from an often cold and senseless, hateful world or society—things that might have caused me undue anxieties or emotional pains, hadn't it been for me having advance insight and knowledge of what to possibly expect.

Another important and valuable thing that I have learned is that not all suffering is necessarily bad for us. Because, sometimes, going through the heat of persecution or hard times can make us better and stronger. It's like the ancient procedure of how gold was refined through fire; a process that consisted of slowly heating up the gold and boiling off any impurities, so that in the end the only thing remaining was pure gold. The same thing can be true of the trials and sufferings that we personally go through—the final or ending outcome can yield good and positive results. For one, it can help to develop strong character in us. Also, it can aid in helping us to produce valuable qualities, such as patience, endurance, and self control, etc—things that might not have happened, hadn't it been for the trials and fiery tests revealing weaknesses in us that we needed to recognize and work on—either to strengthen, or remove.

An additional thing that life's negative experiences and problems can do for us, is that they can move or inspire us to do and achieve things that we might not have accomplished, hadn't it been for us going through difficult and hard times. For example, speaking from personal experience, in regards to my life and situation, I am now the proud author of five published books, which is an amazing feat that possibly might not have ever happened, if it weren't for the negative and bad experiences that I have gone through in life, including having and coping with bipolar disorder.

So if you happen to be a bipolar disorder patient, and you are feeling down or embarrassed for having the illness, don't be too hard on yourself, thinking that you are a total failure or that your life is a complete mess. Instead, you should try to look on the positive and bright side of things. Often, bipolar people are very gifted, creative, and intelligent people—as was shown earlier in chapter two of this book, some of the most influential and famous people in history where/are bipolar. And they have made a big impact on life and the world. For just think, what would life have been like without an Abraham Lincoln, or an Isaac Newton, or a Florence Nightingale, or a Ludwig van Beethoven, or a Mark Twain, and the list goes on and on. The fact is, as humans, both our positive and negative features make us the unique, valuable, and distinct individuals that we are. Interestingly, sometimes the so called ugly or negative things about ourselves that we consider to be weaknesses or most undesirable, are the very things that bring out the best in us. So take heart, and make the most of a seemingly negative or bad situation.

Finally, last, but not least; out of the many things that I have been fortunate to have learned in life, I've learned that when we reach out to help others, we not only encourage and help them, but we also, reciprocally, in return, help ourselves too. Therefore, as of the year 2019, I decided to dedicate my life to reaching out and helping other people in any possible way that I can, especially young people. I'm hoping that I can both encourage and inspire them to grow and succeed. In exchange, I'm sure that this generous and giving spirit will contribute much to my joy and happiness. For the Bible says: "There is more happiness in giving than there is in receiving." (Acts 20:35)

Interestingly, when my wife was beginning to have serious

health problems, initially, she sought out and used holistic doctors and medicines. Subsequently, one day, when I was with her on one of her scheduled visits with her holistic doctor, the doctor, for some unexplained reason, asked to see the palm of my hand. To my surprise, after she examined the palm lines or markers in my palm, see said: "You're a gifted healer! Your wife is very lucky to have you." Reminiscing or thinking back on this now, I figure that I might as well continue to put this special gift to good use, by encouraging and helping others.

The Road Ahead

As far as the future is concerned, I don't know what the upcoming days, months, and years hold for me and my illness. But then again I try not to get too far ahead of myself. I find in my case that it's best for me to simply just take one day at a time. This way I won't become too discouraged or overwhelmed.

Unfortunately, when it comes to bipolar disorder, it can make it very hard for a person to function normally on a daily basis. All too often, all you want to do is sleep. The reason being is because of the all-consuming effects of debilitating depression, which can so easily zap a person of their energy, power, and strength. This is the situation, particularly during the stage or phase when one is undergoing a *depressive episode*—the overwhelming, sad state of devastating lows.

To help counteract the effects of this often highly crippling and debilitating stage, I've learned that I must do the exact opposite of what my mind wants to do and focus on, which is often gravitating towards or focusing on things that are negative and discouraging— things that only serve to further feed my depression, making matters worse. Subsequently, to combat this, what I do is I try to force my mind to be engaged in and be active in positive and uplifting activities — whether it be to do some physical exercise; or to read a good book; or to work on a fun and challenging picture puzzle, etc, — anything that is good, positive, encouraging, and constructive, that will lead me up and out of mentally dark and glooming places, and into a more peaceful, brighter, upbeat, and cheery atmosphere. True, this is an extremely difficult thing to do at times, especially when my mind, feelings, or dark moods are holding me captive in a sad, depressive, low state. It's like struggling to try to pull myself up and out of sinking in quicksand. However, I find that I have no other alternative or choice but to exert myself vigorously; to put up a hard fight, especially if I wish to lead a somewhat active and productive life. But, not only this, I am thoroughly determined that I am not going to let my illness completely drag me down and defeat me. Besides, nothing truly worthwhile comes easy in life. Often, if you want something good, valuable, or worthwhile, you simply have no choice but to fight and work hard for it!

An additional thing that helps me to keep motivated and moving forward, is that every morning before I start each day, I sit down and for about 10 minutes I write down in a notebook, over and over again, a phrase or saying that I personally came up with that encourages me to think positive about myself and life. It consists of only seven words. The saying goes: "I am positive, confident, happy, and successful." Interestingly, I find that repetitively writing this down helps, because it is a form of positive feeding and reinforcement for my mind and heart. But not only this, I also find that it is an excellent way to start my day off on a good and positive note.

Another good phrase or positive affirmation that I created and use, which I don't write down, but, instead, I often repeatedly say to myself, is: "I am Strong! I am Good! I am Beautiful!"

Optimistically speaking, because we as humans are often essentially what we think or believe, I am hoping that with repetition and frequency, over an extended period of time, that someday this positive and healthy thinking will become a permanent feature and structure of my daily mindset and life. Will this work? I sincerely believe so. But only time will tell.

Another thing that can help when the going gets tough is to remember that when it comes to sufferings or any other difficult problems in life that we personally might be going through, that we are not alone. The truth is there is a lot of pain and suffering in the world. For many people have issues and problems to deal with, sometimes even greater than ours! And they are successfully coping with them. Knowing and keeping this in mind can be of tremendous encouragement to us personally. And it can also help us to keep our personal problems in proper perspective.

In my daily efforts in trying to cope with my bipolar disorder, one thing in particular that has been extremely comforting and encouraging to me, that I always rely on and that gives me great hope, is knowledge of the fact that this present life is not all there is. For the Bible tells us that God, who is *almighty*, has something bigger and better planned for mankind in the near future — a coming, beautiful, peaceful new world, where there will be no more sickness, pain, and sorrow. (Isaiah 33:24; Revelation 21:3, 4) This means that the time is coming when there will be no more cancer, kidney disease, diabetes, coronary heart disease, bipolar disorder, and other troubling medical issues. What an incredible and amazing time this will be! How can we believe this? Well, one reason why is because the Bible says: "God is love." (1 John 4:8) Another reason is because: "God cannot lie." (Titus 1:2) Also, the Bible says: "He [God] will deliver the poor one crying for help." (Psalm 72:12).

In addition to removing or taking away pain and sorrow, along with sicknesses, God also promises to remove the source that causes these things, which is human sin and imperfection.—John 1:29; 1 Corinthians 15:24-28.

Although, I sincerely and truly believe that God has a better and brighter future in store for me, in reality, for now, I must learn to deal with the present, including coping with my bipolar disorder. In the process, I find that there are many effective things that I can utilize to successfully do this, even if it is just to a limited degree. One way, is by providing or giving both my body and mind the materials, ingredients, and tools that it needs to comfort, strengthen, and heal itself. In other words, I must daily feed my mind and body positive, good, and healthy things—emotionally, mentally, physically, and spiritually. Another thing that can help is by avoiding things that initiate, feed and breed stress, anxiety, and depression. These are just a few things that can help. There are many more, as I thoroughly brought out earlier in chapter seven of this book.

In conclusion, I'd like to say that out of all the things that have been useful to me, with regards to helping me with my illness, that my wife and family have been, by far, the most encouraging and comforting to me. Their understanding and support has been the greatest factor in helping me to cope with my bipolar disorder. Without their loving help and assistance, I can't even imagine how I might have fared. Although, I'm sure that it hasn't always been easy for them to have to deal with an overly depressed soul—one who often seems like he has a grey cloud hanging over his head, or who at times gets irritable and cranky with them. I'm beginning to think that they must be superhuman or something to be able to put up with these things. For under the worse and most trying circumstances they have always been there for me. And they have treated me with the utmost dignity, love, and respect. I am truly grateful, honored, and highly blessed to have them by my side as we continue to journey together through this amazing, and yet, often challenging, unpredictable, and beautiful thing called life!

Appendix A

Appendix B

SLAVE OWERSHIP

Wikipedia (Last updated May 2019). George Washington. Retrieved from https://en. m.wikipedia.org/wiki/George_Washington

Wikipedia (Last updated May 2019). Thomas Jefferson. Retrieved from https://en.m.wikipedia.org/wiki/Thomas_Jefferson

Wikipedia (Last updated May 2019). James Madison. Retrieved from https://en.m.wikipedia.org/wiki/James_Madison

Wikipedia (Last updated May 2019). James Monroe. Retrieved from https://en.m.wikipedia.org/wiki/James_Monroe

Wikipedia (Last updated May 2019). Andrew Jackson. Retrieved from https://en.m.wikipedia.org/wiki/Andrew_Jackson

Wikipedia (Last updated May 2019). John Tyler. Retrieved from http://en.m.wikipedia.org/wiki/John_Tyler

Wikipedia (Last updated May 2019). James K. Polk. Retrieved from https://en.m.wikipedia.org/wiki/James_K._Polk

Wikipedia (Last updated May 2019). Zachary Taylor. Retrieved from https://en.m.wikipedia.org/wiki/Zachary_Taylor

The Foundation of America

The United States of America was founded upon slavery and injustices towards people of the black race. To prove that this is the truth and not just a fabrication or a mere figment of someone's wild imagination, consider the following facts.

The United States of America became a nation in the year 1776, through a revolution against "The Establishment" (The British Government) that held rule. It sprung from the already established thirteen British colonies that occupied North America at that time. The British colonies were formed from 1607 to 1732. See box below.

Initially, black slavery first began within the British colony of Virginia in 1619. Thereafter, it spread and also became established in each of the other 12 British colonies as well.

Later, after the United States was established and was continuing to be formed, 16 slave states were added to the "Union," starting with Delaware in 1787. And finally, the last one, West Virginia, being added in 1863. Interestingly, in each of these states the practice of slavery was legalized.

Unfortunately, as it turned out, the institution of black slavery in America lasted about 246 years (from 1619 to 1865 = 246). It was not completely abolished until the year 1865. (See the charts and continuing information on pages 218-222)

BRITISH COLONIES			SLAVE STATES WITHIN THE UNITED STATES (UNION)	
#	13 Colonies	Year Established	16 Slave States	Year Joined
1	Virginia	1607	Delaware	1787
2	Massachusetts	1620	Georgia	1788

3	New Hampshire	1623	Maryland	1788
4	Maryland	1634	South Carolina	1788
5	Connecticut	1635	Virginia	1788
6	Rhode Island	1636	North Carolina	1789
7	Delaware	1638	Kentucky	1792
8	North Carolina	1653	Tennessee	1796
9	South Carolina	1663	Louisiana	1812
10	New Jersey	1664	Mississippi	1817
11	New York	1664	Alabama	1819
12	Pennsylvania	1682	Missouri	1821
13	Georgia	1732	Arkansas	1836
14			Florida	1845
15			Texas	1845
16			West Virginia	1863

Below is a list of the first seventeen American Presidents that held office after the United States of America became a nation in 1776. Out of these seventeen Presidents, eight of them were born British subjects in the areas of the 13 colonies where slavery was practiced. Because of this, slavery was no doubt something that they had grown accustom to both seeing and accepting.*

#	U.S. PRESIDENTS	TERM(S) IN OFFICE
1	*George Washington	1789-1797
2	*John Adams	1797-1801
3	*Thomas Jefferson	1801-1809
4	*James Madison	1809-1817
5	*James Monroe	1817-1825
6	*John Quincy Adams	1825-1829
7	*Andrew Jackson	1829-1837
8	Martin Van Buren	1837-1841
9	*William Henry Harrison	1841
10	John Tyler	1841-1845
11	James K. Polk	1845-1849
12	Zachary Taylor	1849-1850
13	Millard Fillmore	1850-1853
14	Franklin Pierce	1853-1857
15	James Buchanan	1857-1861

16	Abraham Lincoln	1861-1865
17	Andrew Johnson	1865-1869

The eight United States Presidents listed in the table below were slave owners. Interestingly, most of them owned large plantations, and many slaves during their presidency, and hundreds of slaves within their lifetime. (For proof of slave ownership see Appendix B, on page 217)

U.S. PREDIDENTS	ORDER OF PRESIDENCY	YEARS SERVED
George Washington	1st	1789-1797
Thomas Jefferson	3rd	1801-1809
James Madison	4th	1809-1817
James Monroe	5th	1817-1825
Andrew Jackson	7th	1829-1837
John Tyler	10th	1841-1845
James K. Polk	11th	1845-1849
Zachary Taylor	12th	1849-1850

It is important to note that although some U.S. Presidents were for slavery, on the other hand, others were not. Some clearly recognized that it was both unjust and immoral, and they staunchly refused to accept and take part in it.

From the information above, we can undeniably see that the United States of America was indeed founded upon institutional black slavery.

Might I add, that those who govern the United States today, did not bring about or cause institutional slavery that occurred in the distant past. But rather, they have inherited the burdensome problems and challenging tasks of trying to pick up the pieces and rectify the ensuing aftermath of the serious issues and problems that slavery caused. However, because some past U.S. Presidents, starting with the very first President, George Washington, were in themselves slave owners that owned plantations (even during the time when they were acting as President and responsible leaders); they are indirectly a big part of the underlying problem of the racism and divisions that exist in America today. Because their poor examples and lifestyles promoted and influenced the acceptance and continuance of black slavery in America. It also kept alive the disgraceful, negative, and degrading "false image" of the black race that slavery produced — a distorted, and extremely negative and hurtful image that has been passed down through time by means of racial stereotypes and discriminatory practices against the black race, which has contributed to them being victims of the modern day eras of segregation, divisions, inequalities, injustices, oppression, and racism.[69]

Slavery's End

In an attempt to end institutional black slavery in America, the sixteenth President of the United States, Abraham Lincoln, issued his post-famous "Emancipation Proclamation" on January 1, 1863. And, although it was an extremely brave and noble gesture or thing for him to do, unfortunately, it did not eradicate slavery in the nation at that time.

Finally, on January 31, 1865 congress passed the 13th Amendment that was signed by President Lincoln, which abolished black slavery.[70]

Truly, the end of slavery in America was a long time in coming! Interestingly, from the establishment of the United States in 1776, until slavery's abolishment in 1865, just within this time

---

[69] I would like to add that although those who govern the United States today are not guilty of intuitional slavery that occurred in the past, they are however guilty and responsible for either implementing laws or allowing laws that were made in the past to continue that favor discrimination against blacks and other minorities.

[70] Although the end of slavery was extremely good news, it was quickly followed by a very tragic, sad, and devastating event. For only two and a half months later, Mr. Lincoln was assassinated on April 15, 1865.

period alone, it amounted to a total of about eighty nine years of black slavery in the newly formed United States.

Unfortunately, as it turned out, the year 1865 was an end of slavery, but not an end to the "false image" of the black race. The hideous, grotesque, demoralizing image that kept discrimination and racism against them alive throughout U.S. history. And, which is in fact, the very thing that keeps them from achieving total equality down to this present day.

The Black Codes & Jim Crow Laws

After slavery's abolishment in 1865, further injustices and racial discrimination were encouraged and promoted against African Americans. This was done by means of passing and enforcing certain laws, such as the "Black Codes" in 1865 and 1866 by Southern states in the United States, followed by "Jim Crow Laws," that were enacted in the late 19th and early 20th centuries. Some of the things that these codes and laws did was that they restricted the freedom, civil rights, and liberties of African Americans. And they helped to establish the legalizing of racial segregation.

The Black Codes:

The "Black Codes" were laws that were enacted and enforced upon the people of the black race by state and local authorities. They were laws that:

1. Denied blacks free speech.

2. Restricted them from voting.

3. Prohibited them from gathering in groups.

4. Disallowed them to bear arms.

5. Denied them the privilege of learning to read and write.

6. Banned interracial marriages of whites and blacks—a practice called "Anti-miscegenation Laws."

7. Restricted black people from accessing public places. These were enforcements known as "Vagrancy Laws."

Following the Civil War (1861-1865), the Reconstruction (1865-77) seemed to help in doing away with the Black Codes. However, many of their provisions were only reenacted in Jim Crow Laws.

Jim Crow Laws:

Some "Jim Crow 'segregation' Laws" that Southern state and local authorities enforced upon the black race were:

- *Separate but equal.* These laws restricted and designated separate facilities and things for black people, such as schools, libraries, restrooms, water fountains, and passenger railway cars, etc. However, these were less than equal to white facilities, and grossly underfunded.

- *Literacy and Comprehension Tests for Voting.* These laws were enacted to restrict black freedmen from using their freedom to vote.

Both the "Black Codes" and "Jim Crow Laws" were deliberate or intentional, legalized discrimination and racial segregation against black people in the United States.

Interestingly, the name "Jim Crow" means *"For Blacks Only."* It is a derogatory and highly offensive term that was used solely for black people. The term was made popular by a white American playwright and entertainer, named, Thomas Dartmouth Rice—a person who mocked and made fun of black people by performing a song-and-dance caricature in a minstrel show, while dressed in blackface (theatrical makeup used by nonblack performers playing a black role). Performing to a song he popularized called "Jump Jim Crow," he sang: "Turn about and wheel about, and do just so. And every time I turn about I Jump Jim Crow."

Later, minstrel shows expanded to include jokes, comic skits, variety acts, dancing, ballads, and music that were often performed by a troupe of white actors dressed in blackface, who caricatured the singing and dancing of black slaves—all done in a state of mockery, to the further degradation and humiliation of the black race. For minstrel shows portrayed black people as being lazy, cowardly, superstitious, dimwitted, buffoonish, and happy-go-lucky clowns—along with being musical.

Ironically, because of the success of minstrel shows and the money and livelihood it offered; unwittingly, some blacks also eventually performed minstrel shows in blackface, which only served to further distort the already highly negative "false image" of the black race, creating further harm or damage.

In time, the term "Jim Crow" came to denote or mean *"a practice of segregating black people"* or separating black people from white people in public places, such as in employment, public transportation, drinking fountains, bathrooms, and so forth.

Later, with the passing of time (although it was a long time in coming), Jim Crow Laws finally ended with the passing of "The Civil Rights Act of 1964."

To learn more about the Jim Crow Era, I would suggest a visit to the Jim Crow Museum of Racist Memorabilia, located in Big Rapids, Michigan, U.S.A. This is a museum that is available for education and research purposes.

~

In defense of themselves the United States Government may argue that the "Black Codes," and "Jim Crow Laws," etc., were/are not in their constitution, and henceforth they are not guilty of these immoral and unjust crimes against the people of the black race. However, the problem is that these practices were taking place within the nation, both in their Southern states per *de jure* segregation and in their Northern states per *de facto* segregation. And for a long time they did little to nothing to change or stop this. As a result, it established a structure and environment of discrimination against people of the black race, thereby paving the way for them to suffer the consequences of inequalities and racism that have become so entrenched and prevalently spread throughout American society today—a solidly fixed, concrete structure, which has rendered these virtually impossible to rectify and remove.[71]

---

[71] This is not the first time in history that unjust crimes were committed against people of color. For proof of this see the information "A Trail of Tears," in Appendix A, on page 245.

De jure and De facto Segregation

Interestingly, to keep blacks from gaining progress towards equality, *De jure* and *De facto* Segregation were instituted and practiced. *De jure* segregation took place in the Southern, United States, and *De facto* segregation in the Northern part.

Definitions:
De jure segregation is segregation that is enforced "by law."

De facto segregation is segregation that happens "by fact," rather than by legal requirement. In other words, although segregation is not necessarily enforced by law, it still takes place anyways.

Some *De facto* segregation practices are:

- Job discriminations based on race.

- Housing segregation enforced by private contracts.

- Discriminate bank lending practices.

The Fight for Racial and Social Equality

The long battle for racial and social equality for the black race has not been an easy one. For example, in the United States Supreme Court case, *Plessy v. Ferguson,* 163 U.S. 537 (1896) decision, the court ruled that "separate but equal" provision of public facilities for blacks by state governments is constitutional. In other words, they are totally allowable or permissible. Unfortunately, this landmark decision had a highly negative and adverse effect. Because it favored discrimination against people of the black race for many decades to come.

Finally, in the year 1954, the Plessy v. Ferguson decision of 1896 was overturned in the United States Supreme Court case of *Brown v. Board* of Education of Topeka, 347 U.S. 483 (1954), a decision in which the court ruled that state laws for racial segregation in public schools are unconstitutional.

Interestingly, counting forward from the *Plessy v. Ferguson* decision of 1896 to the *Brown v. Board* of Education decision of 1954, this amounted to about 58 years of legalized discrimination against the black race!

Later, in time, certain laws have been implemented for relief against discrimination in public accommodations, voting rights, equal employment opportunity, etc. For example, in 1964 the United States Congress passed the Civil Rights Act of 1964, which outlawed discrimination based on race, color, religion, sex, and national origin. Interestingly, this Bill was initially proposed or called for on June 11, 1963 by acting President, John F. Kennedy, in his televised Civil Rights speech to the nation. Sad to say, however, he never got the chance to personally see it get passed. For he was assassinated about five months later, on November 22, 1963.

Finally, following President Kennedy's death, about eight months later, on July 2, 1964 "The Civil Rights Act of 1964," was passed and signed into law by the then acting United States President, Lyndon B. Johnson.

Later, on April 11, 1968, "The Civil Rights Act of 1968," also known as "The Fair Housing Act" was passed, which proposed equal housing opportunities, etc., regardless of race, creed, or national origin. This latter Bill was also enacted and signed into law by President Lyndon B. Johnson, following the assassination of American Civil Rights Activist and Leader, Martin Luther King Jr., on April 4, 1968. This was both an important and timely Bill to pass. But not only that, I'm sure that it helped to reduce riots and calm the nation's fear and unrest during this most turbulent and upsetting situation and time period.

Unfortunately, as good as the passing of the laws above may have seemed to have been during that particular time period in history, they still have not brought about total equality for the people of the black race in general, nor have they ended racism.

For today, we often see that the application or enforcement of them is not necessarily automatic. Because people still have to continue to put up a hard fight to have these laws enforced.

QUICK FACTS

U.S. State and local authorities deliberately created, passed, and enforced laws that discriminated against the people of the black race. For instance, there was: *"The Black Codes"* (1800-1866), followed by the passing of the *"Jim Crow Laws"* of 1865 and 1866, which lasted until about 1965, until the passing of "The Civil Rights Act of 1964."

Interestingly, from the abolition of black slavery in 1865, until these *Codes* and *Laws* were completely done away with in the year 1965—this alone was an additional 100 years of added oppression, repression, and inequalities for black people in America.

Far Reaching Effects of the False Image

What negative effects did the enslaved African people's new identity the *"false image"* have on the black race from the time of institutional black slavery onward?

- The "false image" of the 'Negro' brought the enslaved people of the African race and their offspring an enormous amount of suffering and pain—mentally, emotionally, and physically.

- The "false image" of the black race, which has been promoted and kept alive throughout American history, by means of discriminatory practices aimed at blacks, and also erroneous stereotyping of them, has been passed down from generation to generation to the slaves future descendants, right down to the present day.

- Throughout American history black people have been hated and discriminated against based upon the negative influence of the "false image."

- The "false image" of the black race has become a permanent part or fixture of American society.

- The "false image" has created a discriminatory and non-equal environment for blacks in general in the United States.

- Today, the "false image," which promotes racism, makes it extremely difficult for blacks to obtain total racial and social equality.

Effects of Environment

A person's environment plays an important factor or role or in their happiness and wellbeing.[72] It can make a big difference, either for good or bad, depending on what it's like. It can contain either elements that encourage and fosters happiness and growth, or those that dishearten, teardown, and destroy. But, it also depends to a certain degree on each individual person (in regards to how they view or accept these), as to how the final outcome will turn out.

An environment can produce good results in an individual, or vice-versa, it can cause a bad or negative outcome. And, although we would expect a positive environment to produce good results in a person, apparently, this is not always the case. Neither does a negative environment always turn out bad results.

Interestingly, sometimes a good environment can produce negative results. And a bad environment can produce positive results. For example, a person could be raised in a highly challenging and difficult environment with extremely poor economic conditions that cause physical sufferings to him and many others. Now, although you would think that with him seeing others suffer, in addition to personally experiencing these things himself, that this would have a negative effect and influence on him. However, the truth is, sometimes it can have the exact opposite effect. For being raised poor can teach him to be creative and industrious. Also, witnessing other people's pains and hardships, along with experiencing these things himself, can help him to become more understanding, compassionate, and sympathetic to other people's feelings and sufferings. The end result can therefore make him a much better person, who, because of his difficult or negative experiences, has acquired valuable personal qualities or traits.

---

[72] "Environment," meaning: All of the external factors that have a formative influence on a person's physical, mental, emotional, and moral development.

The same can be true concerning a person who is raised in a rich, prosperous, affluent environment—one who has anything and everything that money can buy—a person who doesn't know what it's like to be without or to suffer want in any fashion or form.

Now, to a certain degree, you would think that being raised in this type of favorable environment, that it would have a very positive influence on the person's outlook and being? However, sad to say, sometimes, it can have the exact opposite effect. Because being raised rich can create in him a selfish, arrogant, and greedy disposition. It can make him a spoiled and lazy brat, who is always insistent or intent on getting his way. And, rather than being understanding and sympathetic to other peoples sufferings, he may instead become unsympathetic and callous to their miserable plight and pain. The end result can therefore make him a self-centered, irresponsible, coldhearted adult, with bad traits.

Essentially, when it comes to environments, we usually don't have much of a say or influence as to what kind we grow up in or live in. And we surely had no control over where we were born. Even as adults, there may be limitations as to where we can live, attend school, work, etc. Often, we are left to settle for what is offered or available. Sometimes, this can work to our advantage, or depending on the situation or degree of negative circumstances, it can turn out to be somewhat of a thorn in our side. In the latter case, for the most part, we usually learn to grin and bear it, or make the best of a somewhat less preferred or desirable situation.

To Each His Own

When it comes to flowers and plants, all have the same basic (physical) needs—they require both water and sunshine. However, what's intriguing is that not all of them do well in the same environment. The reason why is because some demand more water or sunshine, while others need far less. Also, depending on what type of plant they are, they may require a different type of soil, either: sandy, silty, loamy, peaty, saline, or clay. Or perhaps a combination or mixture of these things. Also, some plants are highly sensitive, in that they require very little hands on care, while others need a little extra special attention and cultivating to flourish and survive.

The same is true regarding humans, we too have many of the same basic needs. For example, in regards to *emotional needs*, we all need to be appreciated, loved, encouraged, and supported. However, some individuals require a little more or less attention than others do. For example, it's common knowledge to know that parents in general cannot treat and raise all of their children the exact, same way. The reason being is because each of them has their own distinct personalities and differences. What works best for one child, may not work for another. Also, some have very specific emotional demands, and so forth that they need help with.

What is curiously fascinating is that although a group of people may live within the same environment—*individuals* within the environment may respond differently to the exact, same situation or thing. For instance, one may be completely devastated by a certain issue or problem, while a different person may not be fazed or bothered by it at all. Or they may be troubled by the problem, but to a lesser degree. The reason being, is that perhaps they look at the situation or problem a little differently than the other person does. Or perhaps they use a different approach in coping and dealing with it. Or it could be that the latter one is less connected to the problem emotionally, or that they are not totally aware of all of the issues surrounding the matter, and therefore he/she does not take it so personal and get upset. Or perhaps they are completely aware of the entire scope of the problem, but they choose to avoid or ignore it so that they don't get too involved or suffer hurt. Whatever the reason may be, what it really comes down to is *"To each his own."* In other words, everyone has their own outlook on life or different ways of looking at and dealing with things.

Additional Elements Needed

Just like a plant, a person's environment can play an important role in their overall health and wellbeing. However, there are other valuable factors that are also important keys to vibrant health and success.

In addition to the particular *type* of environment that we grow, learn, work, and play in. We also need one that is nurturing, loving, and supportive. These things are essential elements that all humans require. The reason being is that not only do they help to promote peace, happiness, security, self-worth, and other valuable things in us as individuals, but they are also keys to our overall health, development, and growth—physical, mental, emotional, and spiritual. For example, a flower or plant cannot grow and be healthy without receiving proper care and nourishment, such as water, sunshine, etc. These are absolutely necessary staples or ingredients required to produce a vibrant and healthy plant. Well, the same is true respecting humans too. Each one of us needs love, nurturing, and support to develop, grow, and stay healthy. Without these necessary commodities, just like a flower or plant, we will not fare very well. (Please see "The Importance of Love," in Appendix A, on page 241)

Another amazing thing about humans, is that sometimes, just like a plant, a person could be struggling or fairing very poorly in one environment, but if he or she is moved to a new area, location, or place, they can completely blossom, thrive, and flourish in a different and more favorable one!

Never Changing Social Environment

Another interesting thing about one's environment is that sometimes it can remain the same, no matter where they happen to be or where they go or travel to in the world. Sure, the physical surroundings of each area or location that he or she travels to or places themselves within may change or be different. But the attitude, viewpoint, or mindset of the people within each and every environment can be the same, in regards to how they welcome, view, and treat the person. In other words, the social environment for the individual can remain the same no matter which physical environment he or she places themselves within.

For example, a man may be well known and liked throughout a large geographical area that is fractionated or broken up into small pockets of separate communities. And no matter which particular community he travels to within the large area, he is known and highly respected by all of the local people as being a very good and valuable person—one who is loyal, honest, a loving husband and father; and also an industrious hard worker who provides well for his family, etc. The end result is that his social environment stays the same for him (a positive and happy one) no matter where he goes.

On the flipside of things, the same can be true if a man is viewed as being the exact opposite of the good man that's noted above—one whom, instead of being respected and appreciated by others, is hated and despised by all—because of being dishonest, disloyal to his mate, a bad father, and also one who prefers to be unemployed. In other words, he is widely known for being a good-for-nothing lazy sloth who fails to love and take care of his family. The end result would be that he would be viewed and treated by people as being a bad and worthless person, no matter which community he travels to within the large geographical area.

In both of the scenarios above, the man, whether he was good or bad, rightfully got what he deserved. Because his attitude and behavior to a large degree dictated how others in the area viewed and treated him. However, the interesting thing is, just like the good man, the bad man's social environment stayed the same for him, no matter which community he chose to visit or place himself in within the large geographical area.

Mistaken Identity

Unfortunately, for some people, no matter what kind of valuable person they happen to be, or how good they may conduct or present themselves to others, they will always be viewed and treated as the exact opposite. Why? Well, oftentimes, it has to do with what is called "mistaken identity." An example of this is when an individual or group of people have a preconceived notion or viewpoint about a certain person, as to what kind of individual they believe him to be, when in fact the mental image that they have regarding him or her is completely inaccurate or false. Take for example, a person who may be like the second person (the bad man) that was mentioned earlier. Although, he is viewed as being bad and worthless by others, in truth, he really isn't this way at all. In reality, he is no good-for-nothing, lazy bum, who fails to love his wife and kids and take care of his family. But rather, he is a very good, kind, and loving man—one who is an extremely industrious person and hard worker. Unfortunately, in his case, the problem is that his good name and reputation had been slandered by a hater and enemy of him, who launched and spread false stories and lies about him throughout the entire, large geographical area where he lives and travels.

As it turned out, the conniving and convincing liar painted the good man as being a horrible person, although, in truth, he is nothing like this at all. Instead, he is the exact opposite. Consequently, the end result, is that the man's good name, reputation, and character is completely ruined and destroyed! And, therefore, because people in general don't have a truthful and accurate picture of what he is really like as a person, he is shunned and treated badly by people no matter where he travels to within the large geographical area. In essence, his *environment,* because of the slander that follows him, remains the same no matter where he goes.

Slander, or as I call it "character assassination," is a horrible thing. Because it can completely kill or destroy one's good name, reputation, and character. And, in the end, the important things that he or she has worked hard for all their life (that they have spent many years building up), can be destroyed in an instance of time— literally overnight! Can you imagine that happening to you? Truly, it would not be a good or pleasant thing to experience, to say the least. For it can have a devastating effect on one's overall wellbeing, and also on their family as well. For gone would be the appreciation, love, and support from others within their environment or community that they need in order to grow, stay healthy, feel secure, have inner peace, and be happy.

The truth is, when it comes to slander, it can be one of the hardest, if not the most difficult emotional trauma's that one can go through and bear. Because, unlike some things, with the passing of time, it does not always go away or heal.

In conclusion, the reason why I took you (the reader), through this extensive explanation of environment and its affects, was to help you to see, appreciate, and understand what I and other people of African American descent have to go through in life. The way that we are often unjustly viewed and treated by others, due to being victims of the vicious slander that created the "false image" of the black race long ago, during the time of institutional slavery in America (the false image that initially destroyed the true character and identity of the African slaves), and that has been kept alive throughout American history by means of discriminatory practices aimed at blacks, and also erroneous stereotyping of them as a people—a *false image*, which black people today, as the slaves descendants, have unjustly inherited and are forced to carry and bear.[73]

I also wanted to show you how damaging the effects of *slander* can be and the negative and detrimental effects that it can have on a person and their families.

And finally, the main point that I wanted to convey, is that in order for one to fair well within any environment, he or she must to a certain degree, be appreciated, respected, valued, and loved by

---

[73] As it turned out, the perpetrators of slavery used *slander*, or as I call it "character assassination," to destroy the people of the African race's true character or identity. They did this by falsely and intentionally portraying and introducing them into the "New World," America, as being an ignorant, dumb, and brutish type of creature; one that was highly inferior to the white race in intelligence, which of course was a blatant lie. Yes, the African race was deliberately vilified, horribly disgraced, and grossly disfigured by their captor's, although in actually there was nothing wrong with their character or physical appearance. What a gross misrepresentation! Unfortunately, this demoralizing *"False Image,"* as I have coined or call it, which was given to the black race, would go on to torment them, their offspring, and future descendants for untold centuries to come.

others. Otherwise, they won't be given much of a chance to develop, grow, and succeed.

The truth is, as humans, we all need to have people around us who view and treat us with love and respect—people who value and support us for who and what we truly are. In reality, however, this isn't always the case. The fact is, there will always be some people who like us, and others that don't. But, for the most part, we should all be accepted and appreciated by society in general, no matter what race, ethnicity or nationality we happen to be.

The Farce Openly Exposed

The African race, which was horribly and disgracefully subjected to slavery in the past, was not ignorant or intellectually inferior to the white race as was falsely taught. For prior to their being brought to North America, they were already capable, intelligent human beings that were highly successful and comfortable in their native homeland, according to their own customs and way of life.

Initially, the problem was that when the African people were kidnapped, raped from their homeland, and brought to America by force; they were aliens or strangers on foreign soil, where they did not speak or understand the native language of the American people. Consequently, as a result, this failure to communicate immediately rendered them, to a large degree, mentally crippled or handicapped, and in a flummoxed state.

Their experience can be likened to a stranger or person traveling abroad to and entering a foreign land for the very first time—a place where they had never been before.

To make matters even more challenging, let's also add that the stranger or person does not speak or understand the dialect of the native people of the land—not a single word! But also that they are not allowed to learn it, because according to the local law, for them, doing so is a criminal offence worthy of the death penalty.

In addition to all of the things listed above, add an unfriendly, hostile, and discriminate environment, where the inhabitants are bent on inflicting unjust pain, suffering, and damaging treatment on the stranger. And, although he is completely innocent, they proceed to accuse him of committing heinous crimes. So they throw him behind bars and imprisoned him for life.

To make matters even worse, the inhabitants of the land also proceed to beat the stranger, starve him, and daily force him to toil hard at exhausting, backbreaking, physical labor or work that makes them financially rich.

Well, sad to say, this in a nutshell is essentially the picture (although small) that we get, when we consider the miserable plight and life of the African race that were held captive against their own will in America as slaves.

Now, if this had been you (the reader) that this happen to, how well would you have fared or done under these extremely difficult, horrific, and insurmountable circumstances? Not very well, I'm sure!

Inferiority finally disproven. Following institutional slavery, there came a time when blacks were considered, not just inferior to whites in intelligence, but in pretty much everything. However, eventually, in the course of time, amazing black athletes like Jesse Owens, Jackie Robinson, Althea Gibson, and others convincingly disproved that lie by accomplishing astounding athletic feats.

Unfortunately, although today's society now accepts and honors blacks who are superior athletes, and others who are amazing entertainers, etc., many people still show themselves to be somewhat reluctant, and not completely ready to acknowledge and accept blacks as being intellectually intelligent, in comparison to whites.

Personally, I think that it is both ironic and a little strange, that because my inherit nature or personal makeup, which is that of being a person who happens to be somewhat of a deep thinker, and a person who speaks with a pretty descent vocabulary, good diction, etc—that white people often ask me: "Why are you so smart?" A question that seems to indicate or suggest, that because of being a minority, I'm not supposed to be educated or something. In response, I kindly and tactfully say to them: "I was born with a God-given brain, just like everyone else. And, I too, like many others, like to learn. As a matter of fact, I have an insatiable appetite and passion for knowledge."

On the other hand, because of being educated, I also have

blacks who have said to me because of my education: "You're trying to be white!"—which is a pretty ignorant statement, seeing that education is not reserved for the white race only.

One interesting thing to note, is that blacks have not always been in a subservient or inferior role. In fact, God's word the Bible informs us that the first political power or ruler in the history of humankind was a man named, Nimrod (a black man)—the famed builder of the "Tower of Babel," after the great flood of Noah's day. As a matter of fact, Nimrod held a most powerful and distinct position that no other political ruler since his time has held, in that he was the *first* and *only* "World Ruler" in the entire history of humankind and the world—a person who ruled over everyone and everything on earth during his time period. Apparently, as the facts show in the Bible, he is credited with founding eight cities, including Nineveh in the land of Assyria. (Genesis 10:8-12)

So from all of this, we can see that blacks are not inferior to the white race. Nor is any other race of people for that matter. Instead, we are all equal. For the truth is, we were all created in God's image. (Genesis 1:26-28) This means that *all* humans have or were given the divine attributes or qualities of love, *wisdom*, justice, and power.

The Importance of Love

As human beings, there is one highly important thing that each and every individual requires, and that is *love*. It is a natural, innate need that is built into all of us. But, not only this, it is absolutely vital to our overall peace, joy, happiness, and wellbeing. Without it we don't fare very well. In this regards, I once heard an interesting story that conveys the importance of this.

In the story, there happened to be a hospital nursery, where the doctors were puzzled as to why many of the newborn babies were medically and physically not faring well; that is, except for one child in particular—the baby who was situated at the far end of the nursery, by the entry/exit door. For some unexplained reason, this child seemed to be happy, thriving, and healthier than all the rest. It was a complete mystery!

So, one day, the doctors decided that for several nights they would secretly and quietly hide, monitor, and closely watch the area to see what they could possibly learn. Interestingly, to their complete surprise, they found that the cleaning lady who worked at the hospital and regularly cleaned the nursery each night, that after she finished cleaning and mopping the entire floor, she would stop and wait at the end of the nursery by the entry/exit door, until the floor completely dried. And, while she stood there patiently waiting, she would always pick up the baby that was nearest her, and cradle and gently rock it in her arms. And then, after the floor was dry, she would then put the baby back in its crib, and then leave.

The conclusion of the story was, the reason why the baby at the far end of the nursery, by the door, was happier and healthier than all of the other infants, was because of the love and attention that it was regularly being shown by the old woman. What a beautiful and wonderful story! It's an excellent example that shows the importance and difference of how being loved and appreciated makes in people's lives.

Constructive Criticism?

Over the years, society has become increasingly negative, critical, and even cynical in their thinking about everyone and anything. Personally, I believe that this mindset, to a large degree, has to do with the false teaching of "constructive criticism."

Constructive criticism is the process of people noting the faults and weaknesses of others, and then offering their opinions on how they can improve in some fashion or form—in regards to their work performance, attitude, behavior, etc. The truth is, so called *"Constructive Criticism"* can and has been offered or given to a person in regards to pretty much anything and everything in life. However, the thing that is most intriguing about this, is that it has been taught that this tool (constructive criticism) is a good thing, in that it can potentially help a person in a positive way. However, from both personal experience, and also observation of the negative and harmful effects that it has on others, I have noticed that it often has the exact opposite effect.

What is interesting is that although warranted or solicited suggestions for improvement can sometimes be helpful in life; many wield this tool "constructive criticism" like a sledgehammer to bash, destroy, and crush others, which often leaves a devastating aftermath. In the end, the feigned disguise of being a helpful, building, and improvement tool, winds up being what it truthfully is instead, which is *destructive* criticism.

The interesting and crazy thing is, in reality there is no such thing as *"constructive* criticism." For according to Merriam Webster's Dictionary, *criticism* means: "The act of expressing disapproval and noting the problems or faults of a person or thing."

Another source, Dictionary.com defines criticism as: "The act of passing severe judgment; censure; faultfinding."

So from the definitions above, we can clearly see that *criticism* has a *negative* connotation, not a positive one. There is nothing constructive about it! It is meant to tear down—not to build up. To simply place the word *constructive* in front of the word criticism doesn't make it good or beneficial.

Interestingly, a poem that I wrote, entitled, *"Criticism's Path,"* so aptly notes the negative and bad affects that criticism can and often has on a person. It reads:

It can slay the largest of giants,

Suppress the littlest of growth

Destroy even a glimmer or ray of hope

It can cause anxiety, frustration, and internal pain,

Produce sadden tears that fall like copious rain

It knows no compassion,

It will consume everything in its path

Criticism can leave an ugly aftermath.

∼

So when it comes to receiving "constructive criticism," you may want to be careful or cautious. Sure, it's one thing to ask for help or to solicit one's honest advice or opinion about a matter or something, but to give or allow them open or free reign to completely bash and crush you and your accomplishments is an entirely different thing! So take peoples so called "constructive criticism" in stride. Don't allow it to swallow you up and destroy you.

Growing and Developing
In a Negative Environment

Below are some valuable tips on how to continue to develop, grow, and remain emotionally and mentally healthy in an overly critical and negative environment. Listed in no particular order, they are:

- Cultivate and maintain a positive attitude or spirit.

- Have and maintain control over your feelings and emotions. Do not let them get the best of you.

- Focus mainly on the positive and good in people and things, and not on the bad.

- Have a regular reading and feeding program that nourishes your *mind* and *heart* with good, healthy, positive, and uplifting things. Things that will generate feelings of love, joy, peace, goodness, kindness, and so forth.

- Don't get too worked up about overly negative and critical situations or people. However, depending on the severity of the situation, if possible, you may need to avoid or steer clear of certain harmful people or things.

- Don't get discouraged by the lack of maturity, development, and growth in others.

- Work hard to encourage and buildup your family members and friends. For this will create a strong inner circle of strength that will help to support and encourage you and one another, especially during times of need.

- Regularly pray to God for strength, help, and support.

- Never give up hope.

Trail of Tears

Back in the years 1838-1839, following the Indian Removal Act of 1830 that was signed by the seventh president of the United States of America; Andrew Jackson (who owned a large cotton plantation and many African slaves); the people of the Native American, *Cherokee, Muscogee, Seminole, Chickasaw, and Choctaw* nations were both striped of and driven away from their ancestral homelands—located in what was later referred to as the deep south.

Of these tribes, the last to be removed was the Cherokee Nation. Using excessive physical force, U.S. militia troops under the command of Jackson's successor, President, Martin Van Buren, literally dragged the Cherokee people (men, women, and children) out of their private homes by force. And then, they were made to walk (many of them scantily dressed and barefooted) for miles in the burning, drought stricken heat of summer, and through the dead, frigid cold and blustery winter season, pushing and driving them a distance of about a thousand miles, from the east to the west of the United States; across the Mississippi river — afterwards, to then migrate to present day Oklahoma.

This horrific and immoral crime against the Cherokee Nation and others came to be called the "Trail of Tears." It was named that by the Cherokees because of its sad and devastating effects. For along the way (as they were being driven hundreds of miles westward), thousands of them suffered and died of exposure, disease, and starvation.

Why was this unjust and inhumane cruelty against the Cherokee Nation and other Native American tribes brought about? Apparently, it was all done in the name of greed. For the U.S. Government not only wanted their most prized land, but also valuable gold was discovered in the state of Georgia in 1928, resulting in the great and historical "Georgia Gold Rush."

The Coming, Positive, Future Changes

As imperfect humans, no matter how genuine our efforts and desires may be to bring about a just and better world; we often lack the power and ability needed to accomplish this, or to rectify many of the overwhelming problems that are now facing the human race. Nonetheless, there is no need to get discouraged or downhearted over these things, because there still remains genuine hope. For the Bible informs us that Almighty God can produce or bring about real and permanent changes for the betterment of the earth and humankind, and that this is something that he promises to do in the not too distant future, under the kingdom rule of his son, Jesus Christ. This is the kingdom government that Christians often pray for to come in the "Our Father" or "Lord's Prayer" at Matthew, chapter 6, verses 9 and 10. Below is a list of some of the amazing things that he will accomplish.

No more housing problems. "[21] They will build houses and live in them. [22] They will not build for someone else to inhabit." (Isaiah 65:21-23) This means that in the future everyone will have and occupy their own homes.

No more food shortages: "[6] The earth will give its produce; God, our God, will bless us." (Psalms 67:6) This means that no more, will adults or children be undernourished or dying from hunger and starvation.

No more sickness: "[24] And no resident will say: "I am sick." The people dwelling in the land will be pardoned for their error." (Isaiah 33:24) Yes, gone will be cancer, heart and kidney diseases, bipolar disorder, and all other forms of illnesses.

No more war: "[8] Come and witness the activities of Jehovah, How he has done astonishing things on the earth. [9] He is bringing an end to wars throughout the earth. He breaks the bow and shatters the spear; He burns the military wagons with fire." (Psalms 46:8, 9) This means that no one ever again will have to die in senseless battles and wars.

No more pollution: "[18] But the nations became wrathful, and your own wrath came, and the appointed time came for the dead to be judged and to reward your slaves the prophets and the holy ones and those fearing your name, the small and the great, and to bring to ruin those ruining the earth." (Revelation 11:18)

These are just a few of the wonderful things that God promises to do and bring about in the near future. There are many more.

References

Chapter 1
Bipolar Disorder

1. National Institute of Mental Health (NIMH). (November 2017). Prevalence of Bipolar Disorder Among Adults. Retrieved from https://www.nimh. nih.gov/health/statistics/bipolar-disorder.shtml

Chapter 2
The Root Cause of Mental Illness

1. William Bradford Shockley Jr. (June 1974). Firing Line with William F. Buckley Jr.: Shockley's Thesis (Episode S0145, Recorded on June 10, 1974)". Retrieved from https://en.m. wikipedia.org/wiki/William_Shockley

2. Arthur Robert Jensen (1969). How much can we boost I.Q. and scholastic achievement? Harvard Educational Review: April 1969, pp. 1-123.

3. National Academy of Sciences (March 15, 1968). Symposium on Genetic Implications of Demographic Trends. Volume 59* Number 3. Retrieved from https://www.pnas.org/content/pnas/59 /3/650.full. pdf.

4. Winston S. Churchill (1958). A History of the English-Speaking Peoples Volume IV: The Great Democracies, pp. 151-152.

Sources

(Famous Bipolar People)

Vincent Van Gogh, artist. Perry, I. 'Vincent van Gogh's illness a case record' in Bulletin of the History of Medicine, 1947, Volume 21, pp. 145-172.

Edgar Allan Poe, poet and writer, "Poe certainly had manic and depressive periods". Life and Letters and the London Mercury: An International Monthly of Living, Published by Brendin Pub. Co., 1929 (v.2 1929 Jan–Jun, p.171)

Ernest Hemingway, American journalist. He was diagnosed with bipolar disorder and insomnia in his later years, He committed suicide in 1961. Being Ernest: John Walsh unravels the mystery behind Hemingway's suicide." Independent.co.uk. 10 June 2011. Retrieved 18 November 2016

Charles Dickens (2017, May 28) Retrieved from https://allthatsinteresting.com/historical-figures-mental-disorders

Abraham Lincoln, Researchers believe he suffered from major depressive disorder [manic depression]. In a letter to his first law partner. Lincoln writes: "I am now the most miserable man living. If what I feel were equally distributed to the whole human family, there would not be one cheerful face on the earth. To remain as I am is impossible; I must die or be better, it appears to me." Retrieved from bphope.com. (July 2022)

Florence Nightingale, suffered from bipolar disorder. CBC News. (Updated May 2003) Retrieved from http://www.cbc.ca/news/world/Florence-nightingale-suffered-from-bipolar-disorder-1.366460

Mark Twain (2017, March 4) Retrieved from https://medium.com/@michellemonet/twelve-famous-people-who-were-highly-successful-in-spite-of-their-mental-illness-36793055f41b

Vivian Leigh, Holden, Anthony (1988). Laurence Olivier. New York: Atheneum. p. 183. ISBN 978-0-689-11536-3. "At these moments Vivien turned into a stranger, whom he was seemingly incapable of helping. It was the beginning of a long and tortured series of such attacks, to be diagnosed some years later as manic depression."

Kim Novak — Rebecca Keegan (13 April 2012). "Kim Novak says she's bipolar, regrets leaving Hollywood". Los Angeles Times

Marilyn Monroe: The Final Days, a 2001 documentary, shed some light on her drug use and mental health. "We knew that she was a manic depressive," Monroe's physician, Hyman Engelberg, MD, says in the film. "That always meant that there were emotional problems and that she could have big swings in her moods."

Phyllis Hyman, American R&B singer-songwriter. Michael, Jason (2007). Strength of a Woman: The Phyllis Hyman Story. Jam Books. ISBN 978-0979489006.

Amy Winehouse, English singer-songwriter. Salahi, Lara (25 July 2011). "Amy Winehouse: Career Shadowed by Addiction". ABC News. Retrieved 24 July 2011.

Jimmy Piersall, Goldstein, Richard (4 June 2017). "Jimmy Piersall, Whose Mental Illness Was Portrayed in 'Fear Strikes Out,' Dies at 87". The New York Times. Retrieved 4 June 2017.

Delonte West. Ken Berger (22 November 2010). "West deals with bipolar disorder, gets back on track". CBS Sports. Archived from the original on 23 November 2010.

Mel Gibson "Mel opens up, but ever so fleetingly." The Sydney Morning Herald. (15 May 2008)

Richard Dreyfuss, actor, appeared in a BBC documentary to talk about his experience with the disorder. Entertainment | Comedian Fry reveals suicide bid". BBC News. 21 July 2006. Retrieved 30 August 2015.

Robert Downy Jr, "Robert Downy Jr health: Actor's health battle revealed by family member – the symptoms." (January 2020)

Judy Garland, according to The Sage Encyclopedia of Intellectual and Developmental Disorders, Judy Garland may have suffered from bipolar disorder. Retrieved from thelist.com (July 2022)

Patty Duke, actress, author, and mental health advocate. Duke, Patty (1992). A Brilliant Madness: Living with Manic Depressive Illness. New York: Bantam Books. ISBN 978-0-553-56072-5.

Rosemary Clooney, (1977). This Is For Remembrance. Playboy Press. ISBN 978-0671169763.

Jim Carrey, "Mariah Carey reveals bipolar disorder." BBC News. April 2018.

Maria Bamford , David Burger (22 June 2011). "Comic Maria Bamford will cross personal boundaries at Utah show". The Salt Lake Tribune. "I was re-diagnosed (after a three-day stay at the hospital) as Bipolar II". II" Maria Bamford, American comedian, stated in an interview with The Salt Lake Tribune that she has been diagnosed with bipolar II disorder.

Linda Hamilton, "Linda Hamilton says she has bipolar disorder". MSNBC. 14 September 2004. Archived from the original on 16 September 2004. Retrieved 30 August 2015

Carrie Fisher, "Entertainment | Comedian Fry reveals suicide bid". BBC News. 21 July 2006. Retrieved 30 August 2015. "Carrie Fisher 'strikes back' at mental illness". Usatoday.Com. 30 May 2002. Retrieved 30 August 2015.

Catherine Zeta-Jones, Welsh actress, has Bipolar II disorder. Fleeman, Mike (13 April 2011). "Catherine Zeta-Jones Treated for Bipolar Disorder". People. Time, Inc. Retrieved 13 April 2011

Jean-Claude Van Damme (2012, May 2) Retrieved from http://www.howibeatdepression.com/how-jean-claude-van-damme-beats-bipolar.

Connie Francis. Robert Sokol (1 March 2007). "Lipstick on your collar?". Bay Area Reporter

Nina Simone. Higgins, Ria (24 June 2007). "Best of Times Worst of Times Simone". The Times. London. Retrieved 8 May 2010. "Interview with her daughter."

Frank Sinatra, American singer and actor. "Being an 18-karat manic depressive, and having lived a life of violent emotional contradictions, I have an over-acute capacity for sadness as well as elation."Summers, Anthony; Swan, Robbyn (2005). Sinatra: The Life. New York: Alfred A. Knopf. ISBN 978-0-375-41400-8.

Charlie Sheen, American actor. Charlie Sheen reveals bipolar diagnosis on Dr Oz". Evening Standard. 19 January 2016. Retrieved 3 August 2020.

Jimi Hendrix, wrote a song about his own life and experience entitled: "Manic-Depression."

Charlie Pride, Pride, Charley (May 1995). Pride: The Charley Pride Story. Quill. "Pride discusses business ventures that succeeded and those that failed, as well as his bouts with manic depression. He tells his story with no bitterness but lots of homespun advice and humor."

Kurt Cobain, "What Nirvana's Lithium says about religion and mental health."

Britney Spears opens up on bipolar disorder: 'I turn into a different person' Caitlin McBride in Irish Independent, 23 Dec 2013, visited 24 Jul 2020

Sinead O'Connor, Today.com: "Sinead O' Connor opens up about mental illness struggle in emotional video."

Dusty Springfield, English pop singer. Eliscu, Jenny. (14 June 2007), "The Diva and Her Demons." Rolling Stone. (1028):58–69. Retrieved 23 July 2011. Annie J. Randall (2009). Dusty!: Queen of the Postmods. Oxford University Press. p. 128. ISBN 978-0199887040.

Rene Russo, American actress, producer, and former model. Christie D'Zurilla (15 October 2014). "Rene Russo didn't expect to reveal her bipolar disorder – but she did". Los Angeles Times.

Chris Brown, American singer, songwriter, rapper, dancer, and actor, Brown has been diagnosed with Bipolar II disorder. Miriam Coleman (1 March 2014). "Chris Brown Suffers From Bipolar Disorder, PTSD, Says Court Report". Rolling Stone

Selena Gomez, American singer-songwriter and actress. Revealed her bipolar diagnosis in April 2020 in an Instagram livestream with Miley Cyrus.

Demi Lovato: Bipolar but staying strong. (2015). Retrieved from treatmentadvocacycenter.org/about-us/our-blog/69/2036

Mariah Carey, American singer-songwriter. Diagnosed with Bipolar II disorder in 2001. Mariah Carey reveals bipolar disorder". BBC News. 1 April 2018. Retrieved 11 April 2018.

Dick Cavett, "CNN.com – Transcripts". Transcripts.cnn.com. 12 June 2005. Retrieved 30 August 2015

Jane Pauley, TV presenter and journalist. The former Today and Dateline host describes being diagnosed with bipolar disorder in her 2004 autobiography Skywriting: A Life Out of the Blue, as well as on her short-lived talk show.

Jesse Jackson, Jr., former member of the United States House of Representatives, has stated he's been diagnosed with bipolar II disorder. Szalavitz, Maia (16 August 2012). "Jesse Jackson Jr.'s Bipolar 2: A Diagnosis Muddled by the Market". Time. Time Inc. Retrieved 16 August 2012.

Jonathan Winters. Pat Dowell (30 July 2011). "Jonathan Winters Reflects On A Lifetime Of Laughs." Weekend Edition Saturday. NPR

Ted Turner, American Media businessman. Founder of CNN. At Long Last,

He's Citizen Ted." Forbes. Retrieved 30 August 2015

Ben Stiller, Quote of the Day: Ben Stiller on depression". 20 August 2001

Burgess Meredith, "Burgess Meredith dies at 89 – 10 September 1997". CNN. 10 September 1997. Retrieved 30 August 2015

Jaco Pastorius, jazz musician. "Jaco was diagnosed with this clinical bipolar condition in the fall of 1982. The events which led up to it were considered "uncontrolled and reckless" incidents.

Francis Ford Coppola, American film director, producer, and screenwriter, was diagnosed by a psychiatrist as having bipolar disorder. Phillips, Gene D. (2013). Godfather: The Intimate Francis Ford Coppola. University Press of Kentucky. p. 157. ISBN 978-0-8131-4671-3.

Winston Churchill, Ye, R. (2015). International Bipolar Foundation, "Winston Churchill and mental illness."

Theodore Roosevelt, psychologist Kay Redfield Jamison said she characterized Theodore Roosevelt as: "hypomanic on a mild day. He wrote 40 books, and read a book a day, even as president. He also went into an extended depression that saw him reinvent himself as a cowboy." Retrieved from bphope.com (July 2022)

Ludwig van Beethoven (2012, September 12) Retrieved from https://www.theatlantic.com/health/archive/2012/09/historical-geniuses-and-their-psychiatric-conditions/262249/ (2017, May 28) Retrieved from https://allthatsinteresting.com/historical-figures-mental-disorders.

Wolfgang Amadeus Mozart (2017, April 11) Retrieved from https://graduateway.com/mozart-and-bipolar-disorder/

Earnest Hemingway, "Being Ernest: John Walsh unravels the mystery behind Hemingway's suicide". Independent.co.uk. 10 June 2011. Retrieved 18 November 2016. Thakkar, Vatsal; Collins, Christine Elaine (2006). Depression and Bipolar Disorder. Infobase Publishing. p. 15. ISBN 978-1-4381-1836-9. Hemingway family mental illness explored in new film". Retrieved 18 November 2016.

Virginia Woolf. Dalsimer, Katherine (May 2004). "Virginia Woolf (1882–1941)". American Journal of Psychiatry. 161 (5): 809. doi:10.1176/appi.ajp.161.5.809. PMID 15121644.

Rembrandt van Rijn (2007, January) Retrieved from https://pubmed.ncbi.nlm.nih.gov/17220733/

Pablo Picasso, Irregular: Bipolar Picasso. (2016, October 10). Retrieved September 25, 2020 from https://centmagazine.co.uk/art-bipolar-picasso/

Sir Isaac Newton, "The Madness of Sir Isaac Newton." (2012, September 12) Retrieved from https://www.theatlantic.com/health/archive/2012/09/historical-geniuses-and-their-psychiatric-conditions/262249/ (2017, May 28) Retrieved from https://allthatsinteresting.com/historical-figures-mental-disorders.

ABOUT THE AUTHOR

Author Charles Shelton is a graduate of Northwestern Electronics College of Technology. He lives in the state of Minnesota. He enjoys reading, writing, art, painting, composing original music, vacationing in Florida, and spending time with family and friends.

Other books written by Charles are: *"The Amazing Story of How I Cured my Bipolar Disorder"* and *"Poems That Touch Home"* and *"The Kingdom of Colors, Words, and Sounds"* and *"Short Stories by Charles Shelton"* and *"Emerald Green."*

DISCLAIMER

This book is not intended to provide medical advice or to take the place of medical advice and treatment from your personal physician. Readers are advised to consult their own doctors or other qualified health professionals regarding the treatment of medical conditions. The author shall not be held liable or responsible for any misunderstanding or misuse of the information contained in this book or for any loss, damage, or injury caused, or alleged to be caused, directly or indirectly by any treatment, action, or application of any lifestyles, exercises, actions, treatments, vitamins, herbs, minerals, amino acid supplements, or any food or food source discussed in this book. The U.S. Food and Drug Administration have not evaluated the statements in this book. The information is not intended to diagnose, threat, cure, or prevent any disease.

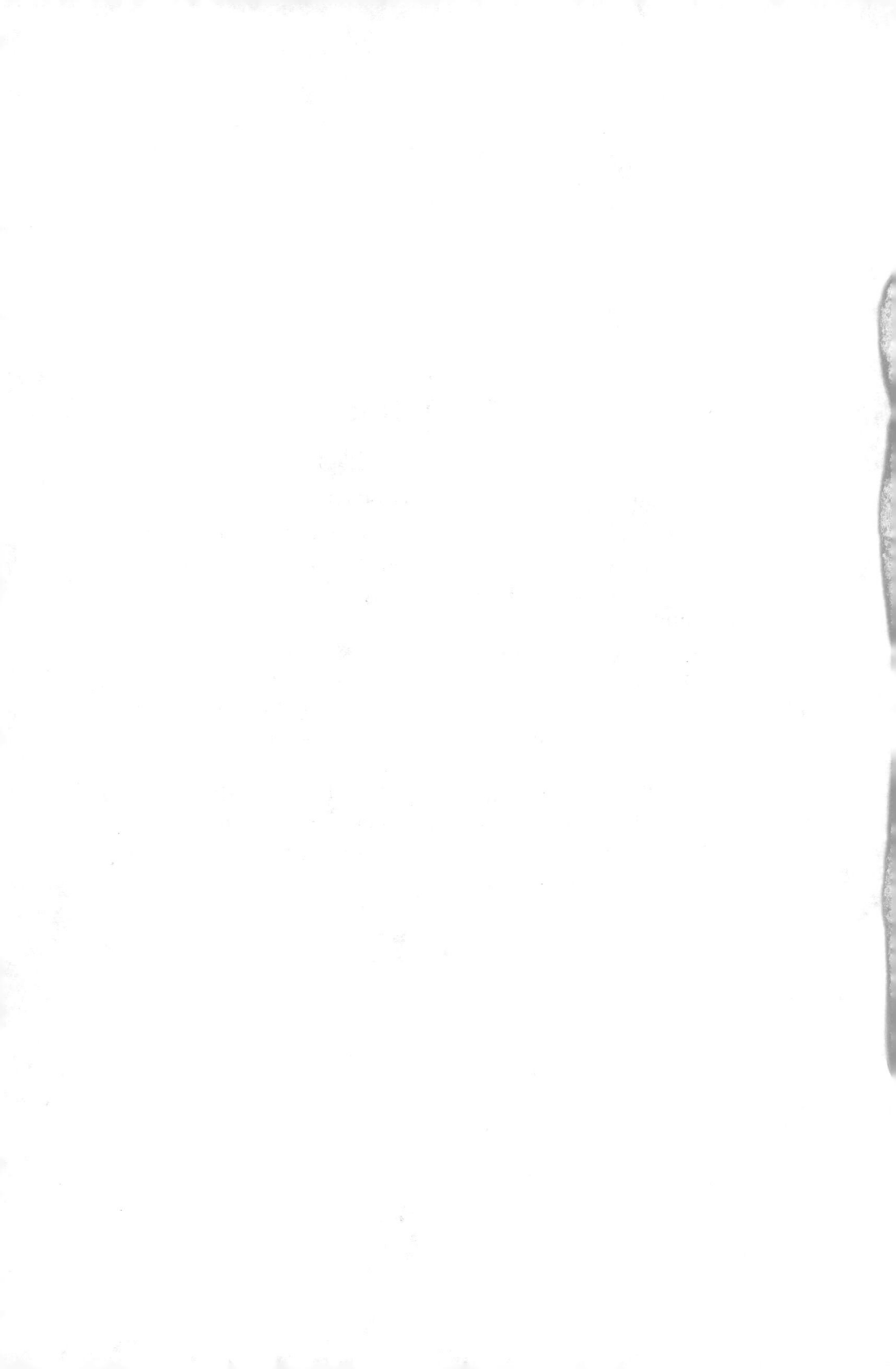